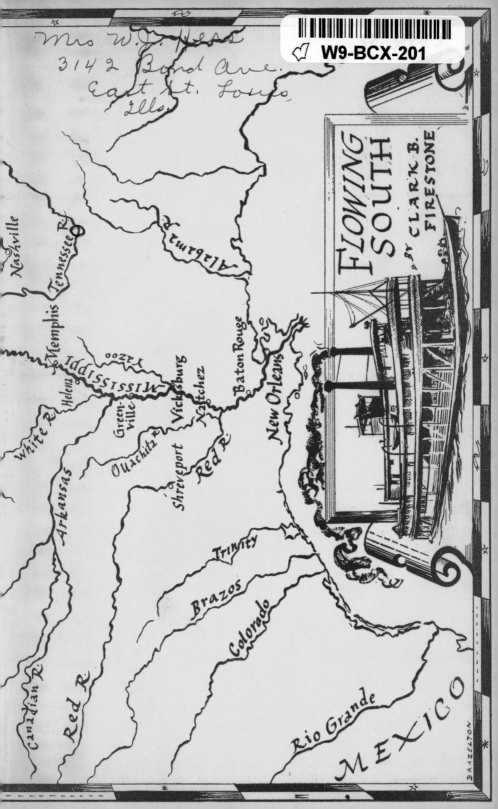

FLOWING SOUTH
BY CLARK B. FIRESTONE

Mrs W. J. Hess
3142 Bond Ave.
East St. Louis,
Ills.

FLOWING SOUTH

FLOWING SOUTH

By CLARK B. FIRESTONE

Author of "The Coasts of Illusion,"
"Sycamore Shores," "The Winding Road,"
"Bubbling Waters," and "Journey to Japan"

"To reach felicity one
must cross water."

ROBERT M. McBRIDE & COMPANY
New York

ACKNOWLEDGMENT

Portions of this book have appeared in the Cincinnati *Times-Star* and are reprinted with its permission. A fragment is from the New York *Evening Mail* and is reprinted by permission of the New York *World-Telegram*. The verse in the chapter "By Care Forgot" is from the author's book *The Winding Road* and is reprinted by permission of the Caxton Press. Acknowledging these courtesies with appreciation, the author would also make special acknowledgment for critical aid and counsel to his wife, Beatrice Sturges Firestone, companion on most of these trips.

CONTENTS

CONTENTS

7

ILLUSTRATIONS

PREFACE

The rivers of the world were its first highways and over most of the earth are still its greatest. Beside them, in Egypt, in Babylonia, and in China, men first associated themselves for common ends and won to civilization. This service the Danube, the Rhine, and the Volga extended to Europe. On the rivers of Africa and South America more primitive cultures have been nurtured.

In belief that a similar picture has been sketched in his own country, the author has sought to learn, by travel upon them, something of the larger streams that flow down its Great Valley. This book tells what he saw and heard and thought. It is about packets with their crews and passengers, and the ruder craft and crews that were before them; about the rivers themselves with their shores, and about trading posts, forts, outlaw camps, and towns that arose beside them, usually where a tributary came in. The tributaries, many of them, came from far places, and so have brought with them some glimpses of peoples, savage or only half savage, dwelling in or passing through a land of buffalo herds, prairie-dog towns, and little rain. On its far horizon is the loom of snow-clad peaks.

Though this record be but as driftwood soon to rest on a sand bar or sink in a backwater, the author is content that for some moments he was afloat upon great waters, passenger on what he conceives to be the stream of time. Rivers are its symbol.

C. B. F.

CINCINNATI, OHIO
July, 1941

FLOWING SOUTH

CHAPTER I

DOWN THE OHIO

THIS was a navigation of consequence. Not in years had any packet moved upon the inland waterways in winter. Yet we were doing what everybody on our side of the mountains yearned to do when the Republic was young. To folk in the haggard frontier settlements and little humdrum towns, and along the dirt roads leading to them, every side-wheeler was a floating palace, and a trip to brilliant, exotic New Orleans, with its foreign tongues and wines, its beautiful women of all shades, its incessant dueling, and its strange beguiling cookery, was something to be talked about for a lifetime. Shadowy packets seemed to move before and behind us, and the scent of patchouli, the swish of crinoline, the click of poker chips, were in the winds of memory, if not in those of the river.

For me this was not only an adventure in itself but another step in a plan to enlarge my acquaintance, so far as might be, with the great waterways of the Valley. Of two of them I knew something already, the upper Ohio and the Middle Mississippi. What I saw of them, though that was before the present trip, is set down later in this narrative. In years subsequent to the present trip I voyaged also on the Upper Mississippi and the Missouri. This book is the harvest of rather more than five thousand miles of river travel covered in five vacations, in 1930, 1937, 1938, 1940 and 1941, together with side-glances at tributary streams which have something to tell, and gleanings from briefer journeys by land and water at other times and places. In

one chapter I have ventured to carry the story of Moonlight Boats into a dim past. Elsewhere I have been content
to pause and look around at a typical river port, which is
my own Cincinnati.

So, on a February afternoon in 1938, we set out from
Cincinnati, which is, and long has been, not only a good
place to study riverside life but the one place to start from
if you are going south. With the Queen City at one end and
the Crescent City at the other—to use the terms of baroque
yesterdays—a river trip opens and closes right. Though the
two towns pulled apart as the railroads brought them nearer
together, through most of their history they have been inti-
mately related, akin in sentiment and interest, holding in a
common keeping the gleaming highway that sweeps down
through the continent from the farther side of the mountains to the Gulf. While one was the southernmost outpost
of Yankeedom and the other the Creole capital, they understood each other.

In the steamboat heyday the people of Cincinnati were
founding schools, forming clubs, starting newspapers, writing books, debating creeds and cultures—and that was perhaps the Yankee side, which led one writer to call the city
"the wild half-sister of Athens and Florence." The other
side, which was musical, came up from the South, and
found a home in the town where it seemed that everybody
was either making pianos, organs, or melodeons, or playing upon them, or singing beside them. There Foster began
writing the songs of slavery. There the minstrel show was
born—Ethiopian minstrelsy it was called. Thence the first
showboats were sent out to play the streams of the Old
West, the bayous of the Deep South. Cincinnati folk-art
went around the world, and in all of it was the sound of
flowing water. One other thing—a book—came in the 1850's
from the town on the right bank of the Ohio, and though

its scenes were Southern it did not take so well in the land it pictured.

I had descended the Ohio before when it was summer. My second journey, in good and numerous company, has left with me a memory of high water, and winding shores monumented with tall, white-armed sycamores, and high framing hills white with a late winter snowfall. In a strange setting the familiar panorama passed anew: the mouth of Big Bone Creek; the hamlet of Rabbit Hash; Vevay where Edward Eggleston lived and Lafayette visited and French Swiss made a good wine; Madison's ruinous boatyards; on a river balcony above them the silver clash of cataracts; the Falls of the Ohio, the other name of which is Louisville; Jeffersonville, where half the steamboats of the country were built; Owensboro with its night-rider memories; Evansville, former Klan stronghold; Henderson, where Audubon ran a flour mill; Shawneetown, which was wicked once upon a time; the ox-bend curves of the lower river; Mound City, where showboats are repaired; Paducah at the mouth of the Tennessee; Fort Massac, set up by the French to guard the mouth of the Ohio; the mouth of the Ohio—and Cairo, often battered by floods, recumbent behind its sea wall, dreaming an old dream of greatness that was never to be, content perhaps that it was the jumping-off place for the strategy that won the Civil War.

Have I traveled too fast, slighted too much, in covering five hundred miles of challenging river scenery and more than one chapter of high history in a single paragraph? I shall descend the river again from Cincinnati to Cairo in a second paragraph—moving faster, admitting more detail, and yet again omitting much. Steamboats steer by government lights (sometimes called beacons) and by daymarks. All of these river guideposts bear names and the names tell you things; perhaps start you dreaming. A novel might be

written about almost any of the river lights noted here—
usually just a lantern hanging from a sycamore trunk on a
lonely point in the woods. A good factual book on the life
of valley folk might emerge from a study of all these names
taken together.

Here, then, are the lights—just a few of them taken at
random but in order—that I passed while going down the
river: Turkey Bottom, Stringtown, Aurora Bend, Rising
Sun, Gunpowder, Patriot Bend, Jackson Landing, Sugar
Creek, Notch Lick, Locust Creek, Indian Kentucky, Broad-
way Hollow, Grassy Flats, Towhead Island, Canal Head,
Fishtown, Mosquito Creek, Falling Spring, Tobacco Bend,
Haunted Hollow, Paris Landing, Cold Friday, Big Blue
River, Indian Hollow, Schooner Point, Wolf Creek, Poor
House, Cloverport, Hog Point, Corn Island, Honey Creek,
Little Hurricane, French Island, Yankeetown, Scuffletown,
Dutch Bend, Tobacco Patch, Club House, Slim Island,
Poker Point, Tradewater, Goat Hill, Sister, Old Maids,
Brick House, Future City, Elisha Woods.

There is also a government light at Cave-in-Rock on the
Illinois shore, and there has been more than one book in
the name of it. While flatboats coming down the river in
the long ago were liable to attack from Indians almost anywhere on the right bank, the danger from white outlaws
was confined to a hundred-mile stretch of wild water between the Kentucky towns of Red Bank (Henderson) and
Smithland, at the mouth of Cumberland. The pirates that
operated on these waters had their hold at Cave-in-Rock
near the head of Hurricane Bars. There in the 1820's, Bully
Wilson, a Virginian, ran what he called a House for Entertainment.

It had a demure past. Zadok Cramer's *Navigator*, 1814
edition, speaks of it as a House of Nature, just above high-
water mark, with a mouth sixty feet wide, an arch twenty-

five feet high, a depth of more than a hundred feet. It was part of a "most stupendous, curious, and solid work of nature," in the shape of a perpendicular limestone wall. There emigrants used to land and wagon their goods across the Illinois country. There crews of wrecked flatboats found harborage. Sometimes families spent the winter in the cave. Thousands of men had cut their names on its walls.

"The cedars on top," says Cramer, "appear to be the haunt of birds of prey, for what reason I know not." Not many years after this was printed, birds of prey were in the cave, and they were human. By false lights, or false piloting, or sabotage under cover of darkness, or daylight attacks in skiffs, they wrecked descending flatboats, robbed their crews, and often made way with them. It is said that Wilson had fourscore men who would do his bidding. If report is correct, outlaws of the Natchez Trace—the Harpes, Mason, and Murrel—used to visit him and were warmly welcomed. I have not heard that his tavern was ever disturbed by a sheriff or by vigilantes. It faded out when steamboats became common. An evil spot it was. But I do not credit all that has been printed about it, because some of the source books were yellowbacks, and because its most pictorial episode of outrage seems to have been pirated from Byron's "Mazeppa."

From a veteran fellow passenger, born in an Indiana river town, a professional man of standing, I heard a thing that the books have scamped. The flatboats, which filled the foreground of an outlaw saga, kept going down the rivers for two generations after the steamboats appeared, and indeed almost to our own time. When I questioned this, the veteran replied: "I ought to know. I have been a flatboat hand myself. I was just a boy, of course, though only a little younger than Lincoln when he took a flatboat to New Orleans. His trip was in 1828, mine in 1885."

Then he told about it. His craft lay at the foot of Cincinnati's Vine Street, where it took on all the empty barrels that it could find. Then it floated down to Louisville for more barrels. Thereafter it filled them, picking up potatoes and side meat at farm landings on the lower Ohio and the Mississippi for some distance below Cairo. When it had a cargo, it set off midstream for the Creole capital. In its depths were three thousand barrels of potatoes. It was a covered boat with sleeping bunks and a cook galley in the stern; the boy worked in the galley. The pilot presided over a long sweep at the stern and had three men to help him push it to and fro. Another hand with a sweep was at the bow, still others to port and starboard.

From Memphis on, the boat "coasted," as the phrase goes, selling produce at Natchez, Vicksburg, Baton Rouge, and wherever else it found a market along the Mississippi's shores. Setting forth at the beginning of November, it reached New Orleans in mid-January of the following year. There the entire cargo was sold to advantage, and the boat itself, the lumber in it fetching two hundred dollars. It was a highly profitable trip, netting its owners three thousand dollars.

The boy took passage back on the steamboat *Golden Rule*. It had to battle floating ice from Memphis up. One incident only of the upstream trip remained in the narrator's memory half a century afterward. On an ice floe were two wild geese perhaps fifty yards from the boat. "I'll try a shot," said the mate, and picked up a small target rifle. A single discharge broke the neck of one bird, a wing of the other. The packet edged over to the floe and put out a gangplank, and a black deck hand brought in the geese. That day's dinner was one not to be forgotten.

"The steamboats never hurt the flatboats," concluded my informant. "It was the railroads that put all drifting craft out of business."

There is a government light at the mouth of Wabash. We passed it at night. Mouths of rivers are important to me, most of all the Wabash. It was just a stretch of uneasy water on which, at my request, the pilot played a searchlight; but it was ultimate Wabash. Aforetime I had written somewhat of this and other rivers of the Old West [1] and it was the only stream whose closing moments I did not see. There was no Wabash navigation, there were no good roads, and at that time no steamboats passed by on the Ohio. "All I know," I said then, "is that the river washes Posey County—'long a synonym,' says Meredith Nicholson, 'for any dark and forbidding land'—and follows an unstable course through dreary clay banks into the parent stream. From flood to flood the boundary of two states swings back and forth along it."

In the following year the engineer of a great railroad took up the quest for me. Setting out from the Hoosier town of Mt. Vernon, fifteen miles to the east of the river's mouth, he wandered over a country that is something like the delta of the Mississippi—flat, swampy, overflowed in high water. Everywhere were fields of corn so tall that he rode through them as through a jungle, seeing nothing much but sky overhead. The last three miles of the expedition were along wagon lanes among the corn, lanes so narrow that the stalks and ears thumped both sides of the car.

With one exception nobody lived there, though there were great barns and cribs where the corn was stored. The exception was a Hoosier squatter and his wife, domiciled in a houseboat drawn up on the river bank. Through this

[1] Cf. *Sycamore Shores*, pp. 178-191.

flat land the Wabash was rushing at four miles an hour. It was half a mile wide, so wide, indeed, that he mistook it for the Ohio which was no wider, followed it in the wrong direction, lost his way amid the towering corn. The tumbling banks of both rivers are only six or seven feet high, so that the country spends a good deal of time under water. At their confluence is Wabash Island.

Always I scanned the outlets of other rivers, wishing that travelers before me had turned into them and written more about them, instead of giving them but a passing glance. Not much has been added to what Cramer set down more than a hundred years ago. Here is his record mainly in his own words: The Licking is a considerable river of Kentucky navigable for seventy miles with small crafts. At the mouth of the Great Miami is a sand bar; here ends the State of Ohio. The mouth of the Kentucky, which is a large river of the State of Kentucky, affords a good safe harbor for boats, particularly when the waters are a little up. Bear Grass Creek affords at its mouth one of the best harbors for boats on the Ohio. Above the mouth of Wabash is seen a cabin, the remnant of a trading establishment, but the waters proving detrimental it was abandoned; here ends the Indiana Territory and the Illinois commences. At the mouth of Cumberland are a small town and a warehouse for the deposit of goods up that river. The town has a post office, two stores, and fifteen or twenty houses. A planter shows itself in the middle of the Tennessee, or Cherokee, just above its mouth.

To this scanty record I add one or two items unnoted by Cramer and most other travelers. The Licking enters the Ohio at an obtuse angle to the flow of the stream, which is unusual; once there was a fort on the right bank. The Great Miami and the Little find new mouths every year or so. On the banks of Kentucky's Salt River, which Cramer

ignores, most of the gold of the world is now buried; in its
waters is buried the secret of a haunting political legend.
Green River, which Cramer dismissed with a word, is deep
and navigable, and was the ante-bellum route to Mammoth
Cave.

I would rather not talk about the Tennessee, but it is in
the picture. Since I went up and down it ten years ago,
things have been done there, and the best light I can get is
that they are wrong. I trust that those who ought to know
are mistaken, but here is what they say: Dams were built in
the Tennessee Valley to control floods, improve navigation,
develop water power. Because a true flood-control dam is
kept empty until floods come along, when it draws off their
surplus waters, while power dams are kept full or nearly so
in order to develop power, the TVA dams can do little to
lower the crest of a flood—less than three inches down at
Cairo, for example, in the great flood of 1937. The problem of periodic, short-lived inundations of the rich bottom
lands of the Tennessee Valley has been met by drowning
them—hundreds of thousands of acres—under what are now
called the Great Lakes of the South. A number of these
lakes, averaging about fifty miles long, have piled up behind the dams. The biggest, which is being created at Gilbertsville, twenty miles above the river's mouth, will be
five miles wide in places and nearly two hundred miles
long, or about the length of Lake Ontario.

On these lakes river boats with their low freeboards are
subject to storms comparable to those on the veritable
Great Lakes—which none of the boats would dare venture
upon. Still worse, if they were caught in a gale or sprang
a leak, they would have no place to go. The moment they
left the old river channel and started toward a distant
shore (as Ohio River boats run for the near-by willows)

they would go aground on the bottom lands that lie under the so-called lake, or they would stove in their hulls on concealed stumps and snags.

In the matter of developing power this public enterprise has been successful in a large way. Which brings me back to the mouth of the Tennessee. The Gilbertsville Dam is located on a weak place in the earth's crust near the scene of the New Madrid earthquake of 1811. If another major tremor should come and the dam go (as it would, for it is built partly on piles), and if nearly two hundred miles of pent-up water, some seventy feet high at the dam's breast and averaging two miles wide, should be loosed, there would be a parade of power unrestrained which the descendants of survivors, on the lower Ohio and the Mississippi, would talk about for all the ages to come—if there were any survivors to beget descendants.

I would rather go down the Ohio more pleasantly than that, and so I conclude this chapter and turn into the Mississippi as traveler in fancy on the low-water trip of a theatrical company back in 1839. There was only sixteen inches in the channel at Rockport; Messrs. Ludlow and Smith, theatrical men of the West and South, had a company of sixty players at Louisville; winter was approaching, and they wanted to get down to New Orleans, open the St. Charles Theatre there, and go on to Mobile. So they chartered the *Daisy*, a low-water packet a hundred feet long, which could navigate a sixteen-inch channel without rubbing the bottom. In the cabin were stowed the officers of the boat and the ladies of the company, and there everybody dined.

The captain took two small flatboats sixteen feet wide and sixty feet long, and roofed them and fitted them up with berths on each side of a wide passageway, which was used as a sitting room. Here the gentlemen of the company and a number of other passengers slept. Since the ladies, the bar, and the dining room were all on the little packet, that is where, at first, the men spent their waking hours. Sometimes they had to be herded back to the flatboats, and the ladies with them, to enable the steamboat to get over a sand bar. At night, when the boat never ran, people were at liberty to rove over the squadron or go ashore. By degrees card games were started in the flatboats, sociability developed, the packet's cabin was deserted, at night, and the men who wanted to sleep were out of luck.

At Cairo, which was reached in ten days, the packet delivered the light-hearted theater folk to the steamboat *Mediator,* which took them down to New Orleans. Thither, ninety-nine years afterward, I shall follow them.

CHAPTER II

TOWARD SUMMER

WHEN I looked out of my stateroom window in the morning, I saw a great river rolling along under a sullen sky. On either side, the flat shores were wooded clear to the water's edge. Behind them at some distance I caught glimpses of gray-green ramparts where cattle were feeding. A head wind whistled past the boat, snapping the flags at stem and stern. Above was the laboring breath of the smokestacks, astern the thunder of paddlewheels. Cairo, at the Ohio's mouth, was already miles away, Cincinnati two days behind. We were on the Mississippi, well started on a cruise of three thousand miles.

Our packet was the *Gordon C. Greene*. It is two hundred and fifty feet long and forty-four wide. When we left port it carried five hundred tons of coal and was drawing seven feet of water. There was less coal aboard when we entered the Mississippi, and of course we rode higher. On the swelling river we swept along at fifteen miles an hour, something more than thirty feet of water under us—enough to carry any freighter that sails the Seven Seas. We did better than fifteen miles after we passed the mouth of the Arkansas, which was in flood, bearing drift from Oklahoma, perhaps from Colorado.

Every stateroom was occupied, which meant that there were about ninescore of us, in addition to the crew and orchestra. Most of the passengers had rooms off the main cabin, which was also the dining room and at night a place of assembly for music and dancing. Above this, on the hurricane deck, was the texas, theoretically for officers' quarters but long since appropriated by passengers. Its name may confuse the same people who naturally assume that a stateroom is, or purports to be, an apartment of state, instead of just a cubicle named after some state of the Union, as was the old custom. The texas on the deck above is, like the Lone Star State, bigger than the rest, and also is set apart, as the star of Texas used to be on the flag.

There I shared with a native Tennessean a good state-room—running water, electric lights, and a shower bath just across the hall. I must add a term to river nomenclature. Though it may never have happened before, the texas of our boat had two stories, and our own room was on what was called the sky deck. In a word, it was Upper Texas, and therefore Llano Estacado, as every student of a school geography will understand.

Our fellow passengers on these three decks were drawn from ten states. Many of them were water-wise, and knew their Mark Twain and the river sagas. A New York banker raided the second-hand bookshops in search of Americana at every town where we tied up. Other passengers were an army major, an Ohio railroad executive, an Indiana judge, a Great Lakes skipper, a young organist who threw in good imitations of a steamboat whistle as part of the Sunday recessional, and a Kentucky dirt farmer who stops his mule in the middle of the furrow when he hears a boat whistle on the river. "We both listen," he told me. Also, there were men and women jaded from overwork, a group of attractive girls, an adequate contingent of young men, and a number of married women on vacation from their husbands.

Captain Tom Greene was the master. The cruise conductor was Captain Donald T. Wright, editor of the *Water-*

ways Journal of St. Louis, who went along more or less for a lark—there had been no Mardi Gras boat since 1930—but who kept telling us the things we all wanted to know. He qualified for the traditional busman's vacation by bringing out a daily stern-wheel newspaper called *Steamboat Whisperings,* appropriately printed on green sheets, packed with river lore, and diversified with old river poems, many of them written by river captains and yet reading better than you might think.

A remarkable woman was aboard. This was Mary Greene, widow of the man from whom the boat was named, mother of its master, custodian of a family tradition which has run with the river almost since the beginning of steamboating. She is the only licensed boat master and river pilot among her sex, nor are these courtesy titles. Captain Mary, a country storekeeper's daughter, has steered a steamboat through a cyclone, weathered an explosion of nitroglycerin, and borne a child while her craft was locked in an ice gorge. She brought up her two stalwart sons to be river captains. She likes to embroider, and she still likes to dance —and I can testify that she knows how.

When we went out of the Beautiful River, for so the French named the Ohio, we forsook Beauty for Power. The Mississippi calls for large words, such as befit its estate as the clearing-house of a continent. Fortunately, it supplies most of them, and some of the rest may be borrowed—for example: the grandiose statement that it is equal to three Ganges rivers, nine Rhones, twenty-seven Seines, and eighty Tibers. It flowed from Freedom to Slavery, and still, as you fancy, the songs of bondmen—unlike those of Babylon, they could sing the Lord's songs in a strange land— awake ghostly echoes upon it. In the Civil War, fratricidal battles were fought on its heights and between fleets of ironclads on the waters below.

The four words with American backgrounds which I have set down in capitals are weighted with drama. Other and perhaps lighter terms the river has, and in retrospect these may be larger. The Mississippi is the River of Levees, which begin a little below Cape Girardeau and run down beyond New Orleans; back from shore and out of sight in the woods for most of the distance, they emerge at Baton Rouge and from there on are the river's walls. The Mississippi is the River of Caving Banks; before revetment work was broadened a generation ago, a survey showed that from Cairo to the mouth of Red, caving went on at low water or high in all but five miles of the seven hundred and fifty-four. The Mississippi is the River of Vanishing Towns; scarcely a decade passes but some community which it is battering gives up and moves back for miles—and the waters move in. The Mississippi is the River of Continental Floods, where the rainfall of a million and a quarter square miles seeks the sea through a single ditch.

It has its own grand divisions. Outstanding are the Chickasaw Bluffs, a term little heard nowadays but understood of every old navigator. They are on the left bank. Once they were rocky islands or headlands standing out of a shallow, prehistoric sea which is now the Lower Mississippi Valley. On them are all the great river towns—Memphis, Vicksburg, Natchez, and Baton Rouge—all except New Orleans, which is not quite level with the river. On them in the Civil War stood formidable Confederate fortifications. Perhaps it was fitting that the Chickasaws, from whom they were named and in whose ancient territory they were erected, should have joined the Confederacy after removal to Oklahoma, and as the Chickasaw Nation made what trouble they could for the North.

Between Cairo and Red River is the Islanded Lower Mississippi—perhaps a hundred and fifty islands from two to four miles long, many of them connected with the mainland by wing-dams behind which the chutes have silted up so that only in low water is their island quality disclosed. From Red River down to the Gulf, a little more than three hundred miles, is what might be called the Unfettered River: there are only three islands. From Memphis to Red River is the Land of Horseshoe Lakes—thirty crescent-shaped bodies of water, each from five to ten miles long, all former channels of the river and roughly paralleling its course over a stretch of more than five hundred miles. In the wild marshlands at the Mississippi's mouth are the passes—Pass a'Loutre, Southwest Pass, and South Pass—walled with jetties through which the river has scoured its own outlets so that deep-draught ocean vessels can ascend it. Once these mouths were choked with mud-coated logs which piled up on each other in a semblance of rocky ramparts that deceived early settlers; the Spaniards called them Palisados and held them in superstitious terror.

Because ships can, and do, ascend it, all of the Mississippi below Baton Rouge is called the Coast. It has a thirty-foot channel; above to Cairo only a nine-foot channel is assured, and not always that. In this area there are overlapping designations, all of which evoke the imagination. One of them is the Bends, which is any part of the river as far up as Vicksburg; the name came in when a New Orleans steamboat line announced regular runs "to Vicksburg and The Bends," which meant merely that it ran way boats that stopped at the small towns. Almost it seemed that the Mississippi sought to vie with West Africa, which has a Gold Coast, an Ivory Coast, a Pepper Coast, and a Slave Coast.

While no Slave Coast was set down on old maps of the

Big River, it was there, and its memorial is the somber phrase "sold down river." There is a Sugar Coast, from New Orleans to Vicksburg, and rich are its implications. There is also the German Coast. It begins twenty miles above New Orleans and extends upstream for forty miles. Seven hundred families of Alsatian immigrants, lured to the Louisiana country by tales of silver to be had there and kindly natives who would hand it to them, poured into John Law's Grand Duchy of Arkansas near the mouth of the Arkansas in the early eighteenth century. When the Mississippi Bubble collapsed they started back, but at New Orleans were persuaded to stay and try again. They intermarried with Acadians, and their descendants live in St. Charles Parish. They grow sugar, rice, oranges, figs, and grapes. That the Alsatians did well to stay is declared by still another geographical name. The German Coast is sometimes called the Golden Coast.

A river, the shores of which bore such names—intriguing or haunting—was the one place to stage the gaudiest, the most inspiriting chapter in the American story. This was the Steamboat Age, of which our boat was one of very few survivals. Quietly we went over waters that in other generations were alive with panting, bellowing, racing side-wheelers. They had oil paintings on wheelhouses and on stateroom doors. The cabins had glittering chandeliers, carved stanchions, inlay panels, silken hangings, silver water-coolers. There was fantastic fretwork on the pilot-houses and decks, and gilding everywhere. In the ornate barrooms the best liquors of America and the choicest wines of Europe were to be had. At the tables were all kinds of meat and fish and fruits, prepared and served by skillful Negro cooks. Before the bar and at the tables, or perhaps on deck betting on a race with another packet, con-

gregated pleasure-seeking passengers. Usually there were
professional gamblers among them, for it was tradition
that their presence on a boat brought it luck—as certainly
it brought luck to themselves. Down below were bales of
cotton, hogsheads of molasses, casks of sugar, bags of rice,
and nearly everything else that could be bought and sold.

Steamboats began running as soon as the Fulton-Roose-
velt-Livingston monopoly of Southern waters was broken
by John Marshall, and their misfit sea vessels—which could
not navigate shallow waters nor make much headway upstream—were superseded by true river packets. Five thousand steamboats, most of them made along the Ohio, plied
the rivers of the country. Sooner or later everyone of them
found itself on the Father of Waters. The Mississippi had
fifty-seven navigable affluents. Boats went out of it into all
of them, carrying trappers, traders, tribute-bearers, settlers,
gold seekers, and troops, and bringing back furs, hides,
gold dust, as well as Indian delegations and broken white
adventurers, In a sense it was the Broadway of the continent, a promenade from which Americans turned off at
length into bystreets—the tributaries upon or along which
they moved to the conquest of the high plains, the mountains, and the Pacific Coast.

Though towboats have taken up the task of the packets,
and barge-line traffic multiplies on the Mississippi, wistful
it is to think of those yesterdays. What I felt was put into
words in these lines by a Cincinnati writer, which I found
reprinted in the boat's newspaper:

> Packet panting up a moonlit stream,
>   Gangplank yearning for a magic shore;
> Captain strolling in a land of dream,
>   Banjo music through a galley door.

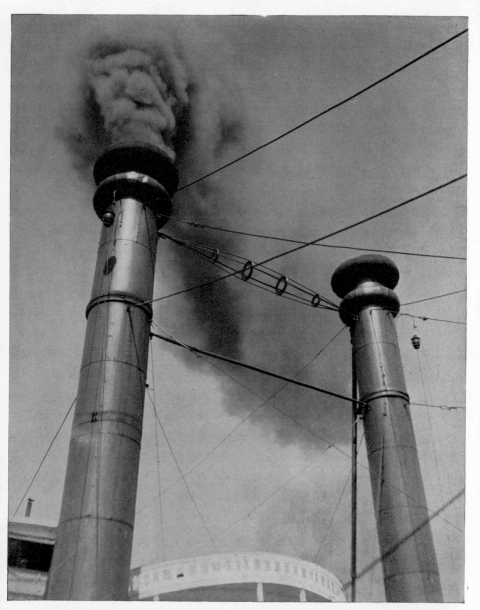

Steamboats similar to those which carried the planters of pre-Civil War days to New Orleans still pass beneath the bluffs at Natchez. To the Mississippi Natchez owed much of its prosperity when from 1817 to 1861 it was a great cotton market.

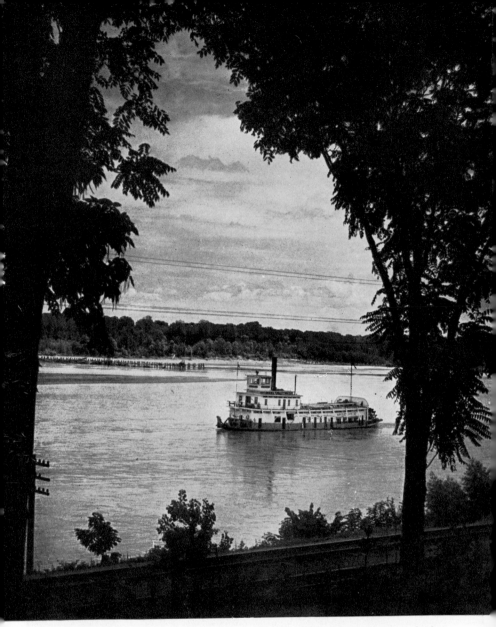

Two of America's greatest waterways—the Mississippi and the Missouri—add to the beauty of the region surrounding St. Louis. Along these two rivers has moved the freight which has made St. Louis one of America's great commercial centers for over a hundred years.

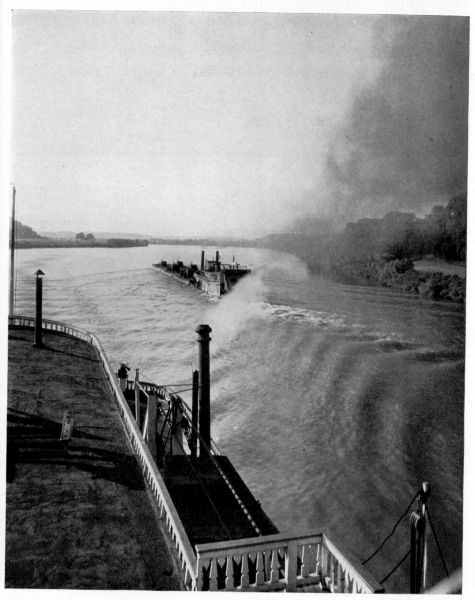

This view from a packet shows typical Ohio River scenery with hard working sternwheeler pushing barges in the distance.

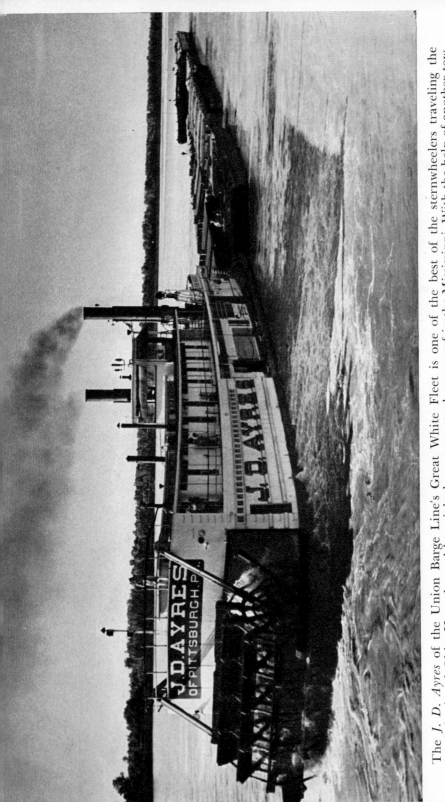

The *J. D. Ayres* of the Union Barge Line's Great White Fleet is one of the best of the sternwheelers traveling the Mississippi and Ohio. Here she and her eight barges are stuck on a reef in the Mississippi. With the help of another tow, she was able to push herself off without too much difficulty.

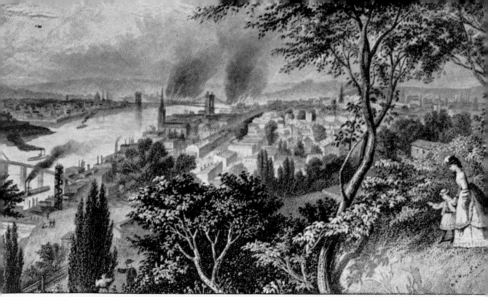

Cincinnati's rapid growth began with the opening of steam navigation on the Ohio in 1816 and the opening of the railroad in 1845. The swiftly developing manufacturing city of the eighties is shown in this characteristic engraving of the period.

The old-time excursion boats like the *Capitol*, here tied up to the Cairo, Illinois levee, still do a big business taking passengers up and down the river.

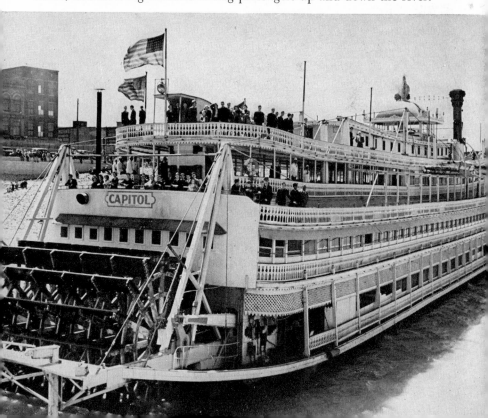

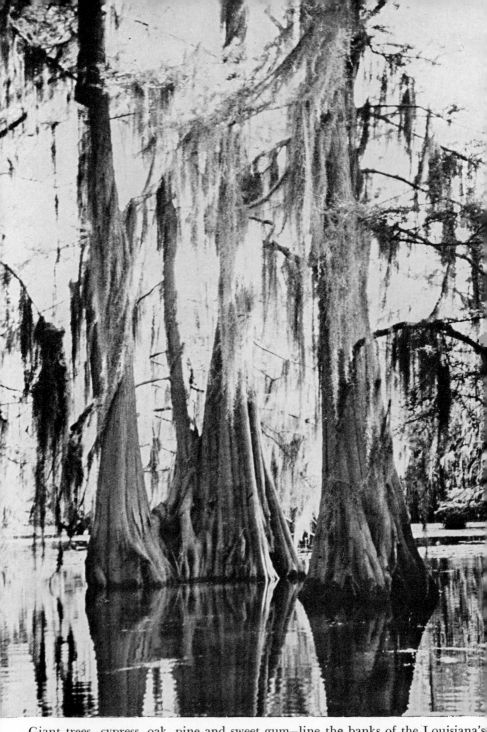

Giant trees—cypress, oak, pine and sweet gum—line the banks of the Louisiana's bayous. Sometimes the cypresses stand so far out into the water that it is impossible to see the banks, and so close together that a boat must be poled between them.

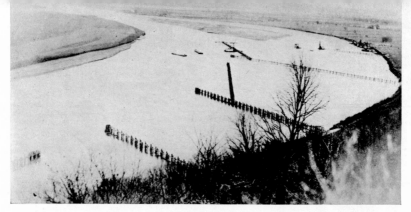

A dike system under construction at Dallas Bend on the Missouri River.

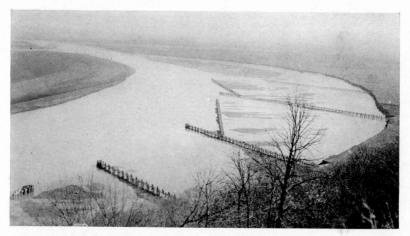

One month later. Note the active cutting of the river bank on the right which has already been retarded by dike construction.

Three years later. Both accretion and the natural growth of young willows have aided in building up the fill behind the dikes.

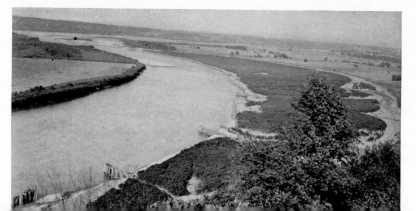

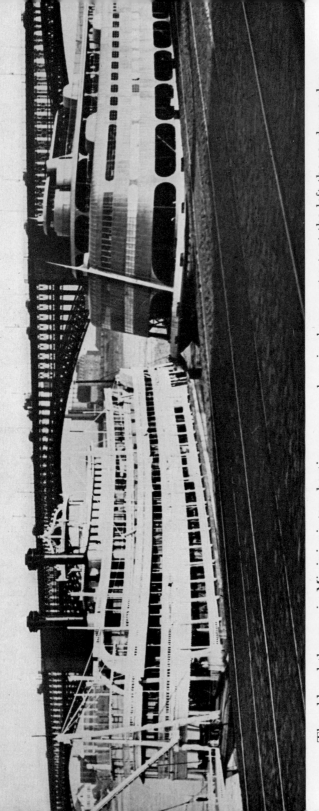

The old and the new in Mississippi steamboating are seen here in sharp contrast: at the left the gaudy wooden boat of the past; at the right a modern passenger craft of steel, streamlined and air-conditioned. Two of the five decks of the latter are completely closed for air conditioning by a system which will also distribute cool air to the other decks despite the direction of the sun on the steamer.

Perhaps the sentiment was shared by all, for we were moving through the past in a boat that would have seemed no stranger there. Save for the use of coal instead of billets taken on daily at "wooding-up" places, running water instead of a pitcher and basin, and electric lights instead of whale-oil lamps, our packet was quite like those of a full century ago, its lines having the same graceful dip and sheer—somewhat like those of a Conestoga wagon—so that when we danced in the long cabin we went downhill and then up again.

The rhythm of the day was set by the three meals, good meals, served at small tables in the main cabin, where dancing was held every night. Betweenwhiles, people chatted on the glassed-in forward decks, indulged in bridge, poker, and seven-up, bet on the marine horse races, joined in bingo, paraded the hurricane deck, played shuffleboard, read novels, scanned the ship's daily newspaper, hailed other boats, watched the banks drift past, appraised the sudden southern sunsets, and went ashore whenever the gangplank was lowered, no matter at what unearthly hour.

We saw New Madrid on the Missouri bank, center of the 1811 earthquake, when the shattered town was dropped eight feet, the well-named Reelfoot Lake suddenly appeared on the Tennessee side, the river—according to report—reversed its course and flowed up hill for a while, the cattle rushed into homes for protection, and "the winged tribes," says Cramer, "came hovering down, lighting on people's heads." We saw Memphis (more on the mouth of Wolf River than on the Mississippi) and its famous Beale Avenue, habitat of voodoo doctors, source of various Blues ditties. Residents of Helena came aboard, and their cars sped us through the Arkansas town. We were welcomed at the Mississippi town of Greenville, once on the river but now, as the result of cut-offs, on Lake Ferguson, which occupies the old bed. We saw state guards patrolling the bank at Angola, site of the Louisiana state penitentiary. Over the levee we saw the roofs of Carville, the only leper colony in the country, and learned that most of its four hundred inmates will not die, when die they do, from this ancient curse. We visited glamorous cities and glimpsed other rivers old in story—of all of which more later.

These, however, were but incidental details in a primitive and vital canvas. We were going through a country which abounded in wild life. Gulls brayed and whinnied about us. Ducks flew up, usually in small flocks, their bodies like crosses crudely patterned by paleolithic man. In flight a regimented fowl, they were easier to bring down —had anybody cared to do so—than the highly individualistic crow, irregular in flight, wary, hard to hit. At intervals a great blue heron, its stilted legs sticking out straight behind, flew alongshore. I saw an eagle flapping through an Arkansas woodland. Far overhead floated buzzards, settling down once in numbers to some gruesome feast. From inundated thickets came frog choruses, the joyous whistle of cardinals, the pipes of bobolinks which early folk called French blackbirds, and the lovely music of mocking birds singing amid mistletoe. When we entered the Deep South, large, golden-winged butterflies came board, and dauber wasps, and yellowjackets.

The Mississippi is the wildest, strangest thing I ever saw. We stopped at the towns noted; here and there beyond the looming levees we saw the roofs of hamlets, and now and then the columned porticoes of a home in the classic manner. But for the most part the shores were untenanted, wooded everywhere—aloof almost as when De Soto first saw them four centuries ago. As always, the river was at its casual, ruthless work, sending tribute by long bayous back into the forests, tumbling the banks, uprooting tall trees, pondering new courses that would turn the old bends into ox-bow lakes swarming with catfish.

Its perpetual duel with the people, whose troops are government engineers, is the most dramatic thing on this continent. Scarcely can it be resisted, though here and there it can be outwitted and made unknowingly to do men's bidding. Sometimes the thought came to me that it would go on and on, taking away land, as once it had bestowed it, until all between Ozarks and Alleghenies would again be sea.

This, however, did not greatly concern me at the time, for winter was somewhere up north and we were moving into summer.

THREE RIVERS

ON THE Mississippi, as on the Ohio, I was looking out for tributaries while we kept on toward New Orleans. The first one I took note of was White River. Descending the Mississippi in 1807, Fortescue Cumings passed its mouth which, he says, "appears more inconsiderable than it actually is," a willow plantation masking the exit. Seven miles farther down he met a small barge in which seven men were rowing upstream. When he hailed them, they said they were coming from Arkansas and were bound for Arkansas, and that puzzled him.

I learned how this could be while descending the Mississippi myself. First we passed the mouth of the White and then, scarcely half an hour afterward, the mouth of the Arkansas. The two rivers use each other somewhat in reaching a common destination. Three miles up the White, a natural cut-off connects it with the Arkansas. When there is flood water on either, the surplus follows the cut-off and goes down the other. Those bargemen had descended the Arkansas and were returning by way of the Mississippi, the White, and the cut-off, because there was a strong current in one river, a light one in the other.

In early narratives the water link between them is variously called a pass, a bayou, or a canal. It is nine miles long and quite deep. Travelers coming down the Mississippi and going up the Arkansas used this pass and first entered the latter thirty miles above its mouth. A century ago the mouth of White had an evil name. At the mouths of Western rivers one of three institutions might be looked for—

a trading post, a fort, or a pirate rendezvous. Murrel's band and others of their kidney infested the region where the White River's journey ends. One old writer credits the spot with having harbored a larger number of outlaws than any other point on the Mississippi. On the lower reaches of the two rivers dwelt the Quapaws and Osages, amid what the naturalist Nuttall calls "horrible thickets" of cottonwoods, sycamores, poplars, oaks, red gums, nut trees, persimmon trees, and papaws. In the autumnal season their country was filled with smoke from forest fires which they lighted themselves to widen the range for game. Buffalo herds roved here, panthers were in the thickets, bear in canebrakes of the bottom lands. The principal food of the savages was bison meat dried over a slow fire; they made a soup also with this as a base and with sweet corn dried in the milk as an agreeable ingredient. Nuttall likens them to "the tribes of Tartary," a favorite figure among travelers of his time.

It was noted of the Osages that they plucked all the hair from their bodies; that they practiced a curious form of polygamy under which a man had right to espouse his wife's sisters or bestow them on others; and that they treated other tribesmen as criminals if found on the Osage war paths, these being designated as such by beacons, painted posts, and inscribed hieroglyphics.

The Quapaws had an interesting name and origin. As the story goes, when the Sioux tribes who lived along the Ohio undertook a westward migration, their columns parted at its mouth. Those who went down the Mississippi were called the Quapaws or "Down-River People"; the rest who went up were called Omahas, the "Up-River People," or "those going against the current." Now the Osages and Quapaws live in Oklahoma, the Omahas in Nebraska.

Despite the phrase of Cumings, the White is a major

stream. One standard atlas guesses its length as nine hundred miles, and some travelers have placed this at above a thousand; the length of American rivers and of their navigable stretches are two matters on which the books are scarcely to be trusted. Rising in the Ozarks, the White travels southeast for four hundred and fifty miles to reach the Mississippi. Light steamboats have ascended it as far as Batesville, nearly four hundred miles. They were on it as early as 1831, when the Cincinnati-built *Waverly*, commanded by Captain Philip Pennywit, made the pioneer trip to Batesville. Commerce on the river is more active than on the larger Arkansas.

At Vicksburg, two hundred miles below the confluence of the White River and the Mississippi, the Yazoo comes in from the east. Recalling that the Declaration of Independence was signed on July 4, 1776, and that, on another July Fourth, Vicksburg surrendered to Grant, there came a time when the Mississippi decided to celebrate both events upon the same day and in a big way. There was only one possible day to do so, and that was July 4, 1876; only one possible place, which of course was Vicksburg—and only one possible way. In a single night the Father of Waters straightened out with a thunderous sound, cut through the ox-bow by virtue of which Vicksburg was upon it, and left the city miles inland. The cut-off created a lake called Centennial Lake, an island called Centennial Island. The island is in Louisiana, which is a wet state, while its neighbor across the river is dry. So there are vivacious resorts on the island and an active ferry service from the city.

That is how I am able to claim that on my New Orleans journey I traveled the Yazoo for a little while. Its course has been diverted so that it flows by Vicksburg in reaching the Mississippi, instead of entering the river as before a few miles upstream. You may call the new waterway a canal, or the Yazoo itself; anyway it is Yazoo water. Thus the River of Death, which is the meaning of its perhaps uncouth Indian name, has become a sort of river of life to the ancient Mississippi stronghold.

The Yazoo is a curious river—in a sense a detour from the country's greatest waterway. In a small boat you can come out of the Mississippi, cross over to the sources of the Yazoo, follow it to its mouth, and there re-enter the Mississippi. At other places, bayous from the latter feed its lesser consort. This, however, is a considerable stream, roughly paralleling the Mississippi along most of the western boundary of the state. It is one river with three names —the Yallobusha, Tallahatchie, and Coldwater—and their combined length is something over five hundred miles. For most of that distance it is a deep, navigable waterway, with an assured channel of four feet or more, negotiable for light-draught steamboats the year around. In 1939 a dredge boat, operating over only ten miles, removed twenty snags, two hundred leaning trees, and twenty thousand willows. An official report showed an average annual commerce over a six-year period of two hundred and thirty-eight thousand tons—mainly of barged logs, with some gravel, hay, and provisions.

In descending the Mississippi in 1807, Cumings also had a glimpse of the mouth of Yazoo, which he reported was two hundred and fifty yards wide. An unnamed flatboat traveler, selling apples and cider, came down from Pittsburgh in 1799. He speaks of Choctaws "decorated with beads, broaches, deer-tails and buffaloe horns" on the banks of the Yazoo, and "at a distance the Walnut hills upon which is a garrison," and that was Vicksburg. Nuttall, also passing by, records in 1819 that there were two small tribes on the Yazoo, one called the Red Crayfish, th other, the

Nation of the Dog, both branches of the Chickasaws, and neither of these used the letter "r" in their speech.

When the Steamboat Age came along, side-wheelers and stern-wheelers plied this river. Gould tells of the *Sallie Robinson* which ran on the Yazoo in the 1850's, carrying two thousand bales of cotton on each trip. It was stolen outright by a sharper who sold it for twenty thousand dollars, pocketed the proceeds, gave a clear title, and went West. When the Civil War broke out and New Orleans yielded to Farragut, Confederate packets quit the Mississippi and sought refuge in the Yazoo, in Red River, and in the bayous. All boats that came to the Yazoo were destroyed, a few by the North, the rest by the South or by their own masters, so that they should not fall into Northern hands. There and elsewhere one list shows sixty-three boats thus destroyed, and eight, including a steamship, converted into Confederate gunboats.

Because the Yazoo ran behind the Vicksburg hills, it figured in three major thrusts in 1862–1863 to capture the South's greatest fortress. On the Mississippi frontage Vicksburg was impregnable, sitting too high—two hundred feet in air—for the Federal gunboats to hit effectively, while its own plunging fire could shatter them. So Sherman came down the Mississippi and went up the Yazoo for thirteen miles, and landing his command at Chickasaw Bayou undertook a surprise attack on the bluffs north of Vicksburg. The Confederates, however, were ready. He suffered a bloody repulse and withdrew from the swampy lowlands lest a rise in the river drown his whole force.

One month later another and stranger attempt was made to get behind Vicksburg by way of the Yazoo. The Coldwater section of the latter was connected with the Mississippi by a winding bayou, ten miles long, eighty feet wide, and thirty deep, which was called the Yazoo Pass. Once the common steamboat route between Vicksburg and Memphis, the pass had long been closed by a levee. The Federals blew this up and sent in an expedition in steamboats which was to follow the pass and the Coldwater, the Tallahatchie, and Yazoo rivers, to a point where it could land in the rear of Haines Bluff, a fortified bastion on the Yazoo guarding the northern approaches to Vicksburg. The course over these winding streams was seven hundred miles long. John Fiske calls it "perhaps the most gigantic flanking movement ever attempted in military history."

Leaving the Mississippi and entering a dense forest of pecan trees, oaks, and sycamores, the steamboats encountered barricades which had been made by felling trees across the pass—in one case eighty fallen trees interlaced in a stream-spanning abatis more than a mile long. The invading force, forty-five hundred strong under General Ross, chopped off the limbs, hauled the trunks clear of the bayou, and in a fortnight were on the Tallahatchie, having traveled two hundred and fifty miles through the wilderness without loss of a man. But farther along it found a new Confederate earthwork with big guns dominating a bend of the Yazoo, tried it out in a cannonade— in which the boats suffered more damage than they inflicted—and groped its way back to the Mississippi.

The third project, almost coincident with the second, to penetrate the forest labyrinth and get behind Haines Bluff on the Yazoo, sought to employ its tributary, the Big Sunflower River, and a network of creeks and bayous. Admiral Porter went ahead with five ironclads and four mortar boats, Sherman following with a division in small steamboats. The ironclads scraped against the cypresses and willows on both sides of the creek, pushed under overhanging vines and barricades, and nosed their way through the bushes. They nearly fell into a trap, for the Confederates compelled Negroes to chop down trees in front of the boats and behind them. Sherman, thirty miles in the rear, marched to the rescue at night, his men lighting their path through the canebrake with candles. Finding the entrance to Rolling Fork—and clear navigation—blocked by a strong column, the expedition withdrew. There was no room for the ironclads to turn around, so they backed and bumped out of the creek and at length reached the Mississippi, after an eleven-day excursion into futility.

Both the White River and the Yazoo show a deficient property sense in their propensity to appropriate the transportation facilities of other streams. At ordinary stages this might be called mere communism; in times of flood it may be nothing less than anarchy. Such indeed are the ways of rivers in the Lower Mississippi Valley, including the Father of Waters himself. A third impeachment may be brought against all of them—a quality akin to vagrancy. On the seashore I have watched hermit crabs scuttling around hobo fashion under shells that had belonged to other crustaceans. In like manner there are Southern rivers that tell each other to move over; that tie up with the first unused watercourse they come to; that trade beds, or take turns occupying the same one. The main task of army engineers throughout a region of some two hundred thousand square miles may be likened to that of the keeper of a Bowery lodging-house who must see that his tenants do not pilfer from their fellows, nor dispossess them.

Wherefore I link with the White River and the Yazoo, of both of which I had a glimpse, a third waterway which I did not see at all in my Mardi Gras journey but of which I did see something on a previous trip to New Orleans. This is Bayou Teche. It is in possession of nearly two hundred miles of channel through which Red River once reached the Gulf.

A bayou is an interesting thing. It is quite loosely defined in the dictionaries as a sluggish inlet or outlet from a lake or bay. Two derivations are assigned for the term itself: one connects it with the Choctaw *báyuk,* and the other holds it to be a corruption of *boyau,* the French word for intestine. The latter, and more likely, shows the same law of likeness as the crude Anglo-Saxon word gut which means, among other things, a contracted strait between two bodies of water; for a singularly crude illustration, a certain inlet of Chesapeake Bay is called Old Woman's Gut.

Perhaps it is not fair to introduce Bayou Teche with a dissertation on hobos and intestines, for it is a beautiful waterway, moving through a rich countryside and carrying the memory of the most romantic of American love stories. Purple hyacinths cover much of its surface, on its banks are live oaks heavy with Spanish moss, and back of them are sugar plantations, rice swamps, cotton fields, pecan groves, and ranks of tabasco pepper plants. This is the Acadian country.

To reach it, I had taken a noon train from New Orleans and ridden west across half a dozen Louisiana parishes. It was a few weeks before America's entry into the First World War. On the train I talked with a sugar planter, spade-bearded, of middle years, with courtly manner and a slight French accent. My questions about the country interested him.

"Where, sir, do you come from?" he inquired.

"About a thousand miles from here."

"And why are you making this trip, if I may ask?"

"I want to see what the Acadians look like. I have read about them in Longfellow's poems."

"And you have come a thousand miles just to see them?"

"That's right," I replied.

The planter smiled.

"I have a thousand men in my sugar mill," he said. "They are all Acadians, as I am. My people will be amuse' when I tell them. Good-bye, sir, I am getting off here."

Not until the last hours of my brief excursion into Louisiana's Acadia did it occur to me that the conversation may have been significant, and that he passed the word along. I shall never know. All I do know is that everybody whom I met in two parishes seemed curious about my quest and kinder than is the wont of men toward a stranger. That, however, may be just the Acadian way.

I left the train at New Iberia and, as my companion had suggested, went to its city hall. It almost seemed that I was expected. A young official took me on a short tour of the town, which ended at the law office of one of its leading men. On the way thither he apologized for his accent. "Unless I watch myself," he confided, "I say 'dese' and 'dose' instead of 'these' and 'those.' As a graduate of Tulane I really know better." New Iberia, he said, was named and founded by Spanish colonists from Florida who cut a way— now called the Old Spanish Trail—through Louisiana to the San Antonio posts. This was about one hundred and seventy years ago. The town is on Bayou Teche. The parish is on the Gulf, whence in quantities its oysters, shrimps, and crabs reach the country's markets.

The leading citizen to whom I was conducted was a judge of good liquor. He led me to a place of refreshment where we had a mint julep—a courtesy doubly welcome because my journey southward had been through a succession of dry states. Other citizens told me that the heart of the Acadian Country was at St. Martinville in the parish just north of Iberia. A horse and buggy and a Negro boy were placed at my disposal.

A ten-mile drive over roads heavy with February mud

brought me thither. After a dinner in which bayou oysters
were a savory item, I met a dozen representative men of
the town whom the landlord of the hotel had invited in.
We sat in the lobby while I questioned them about crab-
bing, trapping muskrats, and the legendary liking of alligators for small Negro children. One Acadian obliged by
telling what happened when a pig meets an alligator, his
final statement a blend of American slang and colloquial
French, "Monsieur peeg, bon soir!"

I had brought a pocket copy of *Evangeline* and it lay on
the table beside me. One of the villagers was looking it
over. When he came to a certain page, he laughed, and
handed the book to me. "Read that aloud, won't you?" he
asked. It was the passage in which Basil, whilom blacksmith of Nova Scotia and now prosperous herdsman of
Louisiana, greets Evangeline and her party who are seeking his absentee son, the wandering and restless Gabriel.
The lines were a hymn of contentment:

"Welcome once more to a home, that is better
  perchance than the old one!
Here no hungry winter congeals our blood like
  the rivers;
Here no stony ground provokes the wrath of the
  farmer.
Smoothly the ploughshare runs through the soil,
  as a keel through the water.
All the year round the orange-groves are in blossom; and grass grows
More in a single night than a whole Canadian
  summer."

The assembled Acadians of St. Martinville greeted the
passage with approving laughter, particularly the boastful

claim for the grass of the Bayou Teche country, which they said was true enough.

That night I slept in state—more or less—in a massive four-poster. As a special ceremony, a small cup of black coffee was brought me in the morning by a Negro boy in plum-colored uniform, and this I drank in bed. Exploring the town in the forenoon, I saw old kitchens in the French style with their glowing batteries of copper utensils, exchanged vital statistics with a number of shopkeepers, many of whom had sired at least half a score of children, gazed long at the tranquil beauty of Bayou Teche, and when a towboat clanked past wished I could travel on it through the winding waterways of an amphibious land. Of course I saw the oak under which legend says Evangeline awaited the return of her errant lover, and the house where the latter, married to another woman, is said to have lived.

Bearing the name of the saint from whom comes Martinmas or Indian summer, the village has a serene atmosphere of Indian summer upon it. In the old days it was the vacation resort of New Orleans artists, writers, and fashionable folk; sometimes a light opera company played there. The parish itself was settled by cadets of noble French and Spanish families who had been appointed to office. An Acadian friend took me to call on one of its distinguished residents. From his father, a student under Longfellow at Harvard, the poet heard the tale of Evangeline. Her true name was Emmeline Labiche, her lover was Louis Arcenaux, and he married another. The disconsolate Emmeline, garlanded with hyacinths, wandered the banks of Bayou Teche as Ophelia by the willow-slanted brook, with "crowflowers, nettles, daisies and long purples" in her hair. So at least legend avers. Her grave is in the village churchyard.

Longfellow changed the tale into one of a lifelong fidelity on the part of the man and the maid, and of her ceaseless search for him—unavailing until the very end, when she finds him a dying oldster in the Philadelphia almshouse; his last breath is spent in her arms. Was the poet's a change for the better? My answer is that for anything written in long hexameters this was the only possible ending.

Anyway, the New England singer has put all the Great Valley in his debt. At the head of navigation his Hiawatha "heard the Falls of Minnehaha calling to him through the silence." Of a genial product of the Mississippi's greatest tributary, Longfellow sings:

> For richest and best
> Is the wine of the West,
> That grows by the Beautiful River. . . .

and that is merited tribute to the Catawba vintages of a Cincinnati yesterday. Of the bayou region of Louisiana, and its "maze of sluggish and devious waters" the poet writes with sincerity and understanding: of cypress arches, trailing mosses waving like banners on the walls of ancient cathedrals, moonlight on columns of cedar, the mockingbird that shook from its throat a flood of delirious music, and wilder night sounds—"the whoops of the crane and the roar of the grim alligator." Though Longfellow had not seen Bayou Teche, nobody else ever did this half so well.

The happy laughter of St. Martinville's villagers when I read his lines to them told me—what I should have known long before—that through the benignity of the years, the Acadian exile had come to seem rather a translation than a deportation. There have been accessions and interminglings of Spanish and of other French blood, and now the Acadians, a dominant people in a dozen Louisiana parishes, are said to be about three hundred thousand strong. Theirs is the nation's cane-sugar country. The postwar resentments of the Old South had but slight hold on them. In 1920 they even sent a Republican to Congress. There have been a number of Acadian Governors of Louisiana and United States Senators. Still, when men of this strain campaign in their home parishes, it is in the rustic "Cajun" dialect.

CHAPTER IV

THREE TOWNS

A YANKEE bayonet was given to one of our passengers while the boat stopped at Vicksburg on its way toward Mardi Gras. The Southern guide who took him through the national cemetery gave it to him after he happened to say that two Northern uncles, killed in the siege, were buried there. This made a hit with the guide, who went home to get the bayonet. It was fair inference that if the visitor had lost three uncles there—or, better still, four—the pleased native would have given him a Yankee rifle, or a sword.

I cite the incident because it makes anew the point that, with the passage of years, a fratricidal war has become a theme for fraternal interchanges. So far as the river towns are concerned, only New Orleans seems to cherish any bitter memory, and that relates to one man; let it be granted that any city which knew Ben Butler as its military governor would have a lot to forgive and forget. At Vicksburg —the first of three significant towns where we made extended stops going or coming—our contacts with the population had a friendly lightheartedness which it is well to record, before the heavy things which once were done there are noted in retrospect.

In taxicabs the boat passengers climbed the hill to the town, and with gracious Southern men and women went over the monumented and wildly rolling siege lines and through a great national cemetery. From a charming young matron with an inimitable accent who went with our group, I heard about Whistling Dick, the Confederate can-

49

non whose projectiles sang as they flew; and how people
lived in caves but got to know the time each day when
overheated Yankee guns had to lay off to cool, and then
they scampered home for a bath; and how the South could
scarcely forgive Pemberton for surrendering to Grant on
July 4, 1863: "He might jus' as well have surrendered the
day before or after."

Below the horizon of our Vicksburg visit was the fading
memory of continent-shaking events.

Farragut took New Orleans in 1862 with a fleet of ocean-
going vessels. Above that city the country on both sides of
the Mississippi, except in a few places, was a low-lying
region of swamps and bayous where defendable Confederate forts could not be established. The exceptions were
the bluffs at Columbus, Fort Pillow, Memphis, Vicksburg,
Grand Gulf, and Port Hudson, all strongly held, all un-
assailable by river fleets and to be taken only from the rear.
By battles fought elsewhere—at Fort Henry, Fort Donelson,
and Shiloh, on the Cumberland and Tennessee—Grant
brought about the fall of Columbus, Fort Pillow, and Memphis. By a battle at Port Gibson he brought about the
evacuation of Grand Gulf. By capture of Vicksburg he
compelled the surrender of Port Hudson a few days later,
the Confederates yielding when the Vicksburg news came
in. Then, as Lincoln put it, "the Father of Waters rolled
unvexed to the sea."

Taken together, this series of victories, usually won by
engagements elsewhere—the interrelation and cumulative
significance of which few grasped until they were complete
—embodied probably the greatest strategy which the New
World has seen. Until Vicksburg fell, and Port Hudson
three hundred miles down the river followed it, the trans-
Mississippi States of Arkansas, Louisiana, and Texas were
connected with the rest of the Confederacy, and by way of

Red River could send soldiers, all the food stuffs it needed, and imports from Europe which came up through Mexico. Federal fleets above and below the two great bastions could not safely enter and operate in the long stretch of river between them, and any Federal army that interposed could be starved out by the shutting off of its river-borne supplies from above or below. Grant's victories cut the Confederacy in twain, prevented reinforcements from its own West, halved its food supplies, and completed the blockade by sea on the east and south with a river blockade along its entire west.

Perhaps no other commander in American history could have taken Vicksburg. For this task, Grant's blend of qualities was unique: persistence, resourcefulness, an incredible patience, shrewd appraisal of opposing generals, audacity, and at the last a masterful contempt for all accepted rules of strategy. Here also, he won by battles fought elsewhere. Meanwhile, he tried everything—running the Confederate batteries with Farragut's and Porter's ironclads; going around Vicksburg out of range of its guns by thrice developing navigable waterways in the bayous on each side of the river; blowing up levees, digging canals, assaulting in force.

He won by keeping the opposing Confederate armies divided and confused as to his intentions, and defeating them in detail—like Napoleon, always having more men than they at the point of collision. He beat them at Port Gibson, at Raymond, at Jackson, at Champion's Hill, at Big Black River, and then crowded them out of Haines Bluff, guardian of Vicksburg's northern approaches. To win this series of battles, all within eighteen days, he cut loose from his base at Grand Gulf, crossed over from the Mississippi's western bank, and with no supplies save what his men could carry in their knapsacks, he lived on the country—too little bread, too many fried chickens! At the end, Pemberton, Confederate commander, driven from the field, was back in Vicksburg, unaware, until a message came from his more sagacious associate Johnston, that his capture was certain unless he abandoned that stronghold. But the road of escape was already closed. Part of Grant's command—now swelled to seventy thousand—kept Johnston at a distance. The siege was on.

Under shelling from the ironclads in front and the army in the rear, the inhabitants were driven to live in caves hollowed in the bluffs. Vicksburg, still impregnable against direct assault, was starved out. Flour brought ten dollars a pound, people ate mule meat. On July 4th, 1863, Pemberton gave it up, surrendering more men than any commander in modern warfare up to that time, more even—as Fiske points out—than yielded to Napoleon at Ulm in 1805. The thirty-seven thousand who laid down their arms at Vicksburg, added to twelve thousand who had been captured or put out of action in the five preceding battles, made a total just equal to the force with which Grant began the campaign.

On the very day of Vicksburg's fall, the Confederates lost at Gettysburg. The rest of their gallant and vain story is a recessional.

Romantic as is the story of Natchez where our packet stopped for most of a day, and beautiful beyond any picture we had formed of it as is Natchez-on-the-Hill, its singular title to remembrance is that an ancient and evil trail ran through it, to which it gave its name. The trail was beaten as soon as there were settlers in any number in the Old West.

They took their produce—mainly corn, whisky, hams, bacon, and peach brandy—down the rivers in flatboats to

New Orleans, the only available market. This was one-way traffic, for flatboats could not go upstream, nor of course could commodities. The large growers, merchants, and speculators sold what they had for gold, and rode back over a path along the left bank of the Mississippi, carrying the gold in belts or in their saddlebags. Below Natchez, some two hundred miles above the Creole capital, the path ran through territory which at first was Spanish, was fairly well settled and policed, and safe enough. It had no name. Above Natchez, which from 1793 on was American, it was called the Natchez Trace. This vague path amid canebrakes, cypress swamps, and the primeval forest, trended northeast through the Choctaw and Chickasaw country, through what afterward became the States of Mississippi and Tennessee to Nashville, perhaps five hundred miles.

Along it singly, or with one or two companions, or in small parties, men rode northward, and each had on his person hundreds of dollars in gold, often a thousand dollars or more. What they carried, together with the loneliness of the path, set the stage for highway robbers. These were of a kind unknown since certain fearsome annals of the Middle Ages. I have read accounts of their exploits compiled from earlier and dubious chronicles which mixed up both geography and history and yet, like the paperbacks of the old-time literature of roguery, had a wide popular sale. Making all discounts, what is left is a disturbing phenomenon even when viewed from the perspective of a hundred years.

There were werewolves on the Natchez Trace, human only in form and at intervals. The wilderness did to them what it had done to men before. Just a hint of this is in Roosevelt's *Winning of the West,* in a passage about white men who disappeared from the frontier settlements, joined Indian bands, and, smearing themselves with charcoal and vermilion, descended with their savage hosts on their own neighbors in an orgy of bloodshed and torture—reappearing later as white citizens to condole with the survivors.

Medieval tradition had it that sorcerers took on the form of wolves just before they vanished in the wood. Those who thought they had this power were madmen—their disease is called lycanthropy. Reading the story of Big Harpe and Little Harpe, of Joseph Hare, Samuel Mason, John A. Murrel, and their immediate followers, one gets the picture of intermittent madness. They were maniacs and openly avowed it, or betrayed it by their ravings when trapped and imprisoned. When unmasked they were treated in the settlement courts, or by improvised roadside tribunals, like wild beasts, which is what they were.

The old English term "wolf's head" is in point. One of the robbers was beheaded and his grinning skull, affixed for years on a pole, gave a name to Harpe's Head, across the Ohio in Kentucky from Cave-in-Rock. This was a resort of river thieves and outlaws who, it is said, cast Big Harpe out from their wild confraternity because they felt he was not human. Little Harpe reappeared later on the Natchez Trace, or rather his head did, incased in a ball of blue clay to arrest putrefaction until the reward could be claimed. As for the others, they were put in the pillory, publicly whipped, branded, and jailed—or, as in most cases, incontinently hanged by what might be called Courts of Vigilance.

Their inhuman nature declared itself in their deeds. Garbed as Indians they robbed and murdered, libeling the peaceable Choctaw and Chickasaw nations to which they professed to belong. Usually they killed the men they robbed. What followed was lycanthropic. The body of the victim was disemboweled, stones, gravel, and sand were poured into the cavity, and the weighted carcass was sunk in the nearest stream or swamp. It is quite in the werewolf picture that on occasion the miscreants wore broadcloth on the Trace, mingled at intervals with the fashionable society of the river towns, purported at times to be liberators of slaves—instead of the "nigger stealers" that they were—and as such corresponded with Northern Abolitionists. For a final touch, the robbers used to don the garb of Methodist preachers, travel with a Bible in hand, deliver rousing sermons, conduct exciting revivals in the woods, and, as opportunity provided, pass counterfeit money off on the worshipers.

Murrel, chief outlaw figure on the Natchez Trace, dreamed of freeing and arming the blacks, assigning them white leaders from his gang followers, giving each Negro a captured white woman for his consort, and with his slave army ravaging the Lower Mississippi Valley. Christmas Day of 1835 was appointed for the uprising; the date was shifted to the ensuing Fourth of July; and on that date mobs rioted—though without avail—in the vicious little settlements that lay below the bluffs on which stood the chief river towns.

The outlaws of the Trace were by-products of slow, one-way navigation and of unbalanced commercial exchanges. It was left to the gamblers, sporting women, and liquor vendors of New Orleans to restore the balance. Thither the outlaws carried the gold of their victims; after a short interval of uproarious but gilded living, the Creole city had it all again. Not the law nor the vigilantes ended the reign of violence on land and on water. When steamboats grew common, people who went down to New Orleans came back upon them, and the stuffs of Europe came back with them. Gold no longer rode horseback on the Natchez Trace.

Natchez itself has—or had—two faces, and knows the Mississippi both as enemy and friend. Natchez-under-the-Hill is now Natchez under the river, only half a score of old brick, verandahed houses remaining of the wickedest little settlement of the Great Valley in the flatboat era. With gray, casual hand, the river wiped out the underworld's undertown, and the hectic habitations of thieves, harlots, bar-flies, and rowdies tumbled into its oblivious waters.

There were such settlements also under the Chickasaw Bluffs at Vicksburg and Memphis, not so clearly recalled because they were perhaps a shade less flagrant, and because the river did not deign to make itself their sexton; Father Time did them under. Flatboatmen were wont to lay up there, waiting for the high, swift water of the breaking spring to take them onward. They had plenty of courage and they could work hard—and that was about all. Of their recklessness and lawlessness, their ruffianly bearing and outrageous jocularities, a hundred books bear a testimony which need not be repeated here. In a word, they were primitive Children of the River, wildfowl such as running water always breeds. The mission of the shanty town under the bluffs was to pluck them.

For the most part its denizens were the scum of humanity, parasites all, who preyed on the weaknesses of the flatboatmen, robbed them while entertaining them, and killed them when it was worth while and seemed to be safe. Sometimes these nether folk stormed the heights and carried riot through the orderly streets of towns above them which made a habit, and a merit, of ignoring their existence. There were reprisals, citizens rounding up and roughhousing the intrusive strumpets; waging periodical wars on gambling, and lynching a handful or so of the professionals. Once the rowdies under the Vicksburg heights, and in Pinch-Gut below the brow of Memphis, joined with

the river-fronters of Natchez-under-the-Hill in a concerted
move to burn the towns above them. They had no leader
and got nowhere, for Murrel, outlaw in chief who planned
this thing, was in prison.

The best account of Natchez-under-the-Hill is by Timothy Flint, who saw it in the 1820's. A thousand boats lay at
the landing—scows, bateaux, Kentucky broadhorns, barges,
huge roofed flatboats, and rafts that had sheds upon them.
The town itself was "full of boatmen, mulattoes, houses of
ill fame and their wretched tenants, in short the refuse of
the world." There were two long streets parallel with the
river and numerous alleys that connected them. The buildings that fronted on the streets were liquor shops, gambling houses, disorderly dance halls. From them came
drunken shouts, the click of crooked dice, the thin tones
of rickety pianos. From alley windows scantily garbed
women of all colors and shades of color called and beck-
oned. The jangle of doorbells as men came and went there
made a sort of eager hymn to Venus.

While Natchez-under-the-Hill, most of it, tumbled into
the river in the big flood of 1840, Natchez-on-the-Hill, as
I saw it, is very much as it was when Flint pictured it,
though more than twice as populous, and more than a century older. He found it a town with broad streets, with "an
appearance of comfort and opulence, a charming aspect of
quietness and repose." Some of the planters were wealthy
and these received accredited strangers "kindly." Their
wealth came from the cotton fields; with bales of cotton
during the shipment season the streets were "almost barri-
caded."

Here, two hundred feet above the squalid remains of its
profane consort—through which gentlewomen passed veiled
when they went to and from the steamboats—Natchez-on-

the-Hill keeps alive the memories of the Old South. Indeed, it is the Old South, a thing which I had doubted profoundly until my own eyes confirmed it. Natchez is of Spanish origin, is older than New Orleans, and has been under six flags. Because it is high, healthful, and safe from the water, safer than most regions of lower levels from the periodic scourges of yellow fever, the cotton planters of the Mississippi Valley built luxurious homes here. Perhaps thirty of the finest of these are still standing, all bearing names, and some of them we were privileged to enter. They are in spacious grounds with carriageways lined with crepe myrtles, shadowed by palms and live oaks, by sweet-olive trees and lacquer-leaved magnolias. They are draped with Spanish moss, beautiful even in February with their blooming wistaria, azalea, japonica, Cape jasmine, white iris, and camellia, thrilling with mockingbird song.

Box hedges framed the walks. One dwelling had a brick-walled formal garden in a dry bayou carpeted with pine needles and a blue-tiled courtyard with great blue-green porcelain jars. Over all was the heavy fragrance of the pride of China and of locust trees in blossom.

Cotton was king indeed when the planters built those homes and endowed them with wide halls, high ceilings, flanking galleries, winding staircases, hardwood floors, imported furniture and tapestries, and ample slave quarters connecting by covered passages. One planter chartered a ship to bring over his great, gilt-framed mirrors and mahogany tables, sideboards and four-posters, and with them a party of skilled Italian woodworkers. These homes went nearly unscathed through the ravage of war, Natchez being subjected only to what the Southern lady who showed us around called "one rather gentlemanly bombardment" from the river—for which there had been some provocation.

"I can see Scarlett O'Hara descending that winding staircase," said a girl in our party, and thereby said all. What
all of us saw were Georgian houses with fluted Doric columns; hospitable twin doorways with fanlights; hanging
balconies of wrought iron; sculptured mantelpieces fashioned abroad of gray, rose, green, gold-flecked, black, or
white marbles. There were banqueting tables set with crystal, and silver services made to order from Spanish silver
dollars; tall candlesticks of Sheffield plate; carved Renais-
sance cabinets; Aubusson carpets, china based upon a bird
design by Audubon. In original pieces of furniture one
could recognize the handiwork of Chippendale, Hepple-
white, Duncan Phyffe, and Sheraton.

Through a Natchez enterprise called the Garden Pilgrimage these homes have been preserved as showpieces of
the South of Swords and Roses. We were weeks ahead of the
annual pilgrimage, when open-air tableaux are given, and
in the pictorial garb of the ante-bellum time the hostesses
of these mansions receive visitors. As a gesture of courtesy
to our own river pilgrimage several of these gracious women
and their daughters arrayed themselves in crinoline, wore
elaborately curled coiffures, and bedecked themselves with
family heirlooms such as neck-chains, lockets, stomachers,
and cameo brooches. One of the women, whose crinoline
billowed over the sides of the tapestried armchair where
she sat enthroned, and whose white-encased ankles were
delightfully trim and somewhat in evidence, made so engaging a picture that as our party crossed the threshold on
the way out I turned back and made a proposition.

"Suppose," I said, "we sit for a while before that coal
fire in the adjoining room, and talk things over."

Her eyes lighted amusedly, and she seemed to assent.

"That would be wonderful," she said, "no matter if you
missed your boat!"

"Why bring that up?" I rejoined.

So for a space we fenced back and forth, each of us quite aware that both of us were fooling. I caught the boat all right, and went with it down to Baton Rouge.

Going ashore at Baton Rouge was important to all of us, for then we set foot on the soil of Louisiana. It is not as other states. Instead of counties it has parishes. Its beginnings were Latin rather than Anglo-Saxon or Dutch. French is still widely spoken and in at least three dialects: New Orleans French, which is more or less Parisian; Acadian French, which is a mellow, rustic tongue; and Gombo French, the still softer speech of Negroes whose forebears had Creole proprietors. The older and better architecture, however, is Spanish, for sometimes the province had such masters, and whatever their failings the vanished hidalgos knew how to rear stately and spacious buildings that would not yield readily to the siege of years.

About Louisiana, as about no other state, both the Mississippi and the Gulf weave the spells of moving water. In the Barataria coast region it has traditions of "Spanish sailors with bearded lips," pirate folk of every other race; and these memories it would not forego. It is the Bayou State, with long reaches of clear brown water capable of flowing in either direction, or of standing still; with great cypress swamps haunted by the alligator and pelican; with lakes that once were ox-bow bends of the vagrant river, and with other lakes, like Pontchartrain and Maurepas, that lie just inside the blue rim of the coast. It grows rice and oranges and sugar cane, and sends to all countries the vigorous syrup called New Orleans molasses. It traps muskrats, millions of skins a year. Shrimping fleets and oyster craft animate its coasts, and out of salt water are taken tarpon, amber jack, and sea turtles, sheepshead, redfish and mullet. Framing its streams and swamps, and every path that leads in to a plantation—framing Louisiana itself—is the gray Spanish moss, which hangs like stage draperies and gives the state a theatrical though somewhat somber aspect.

Baton Rouge stands on the Mississippi's last hill; everything below it, as well as much above it, was once the Gulf of Mexico. Its French name, which means Red Stick, was given it by Bienville because, as he recites, "on the bank were many cabins covered with palmetto leaves, and a Maypole without branches, reddened with severed heads of fish and beasts attached as a sacrifice." This, of course, was a totem pole, the name related to Canada's weather-breeding Medicine Hat and New York's Painted Post. Baton Rouge has its palm trees still. A wind from the south breathed through them as I walked in the balmy sunshine along streets of white, double-galleried dwellings.

The town has ancient backgrounds, stormy recollections of only yesterday, present significances. One of the earliest French settlements, it has been under seven flags, including the banner of the ill-fated West Florida Republic, product of a short-lived rebellion. It witnessed the only Revolutionary battle fought on Louisiana soil. In the Civil War it was held in turn by Confederate and Federal troops and was the scene of a savage engagement between them. It was the home of Zachary Taylor, and briefly of the prewar William Tecumseh Sherman.

On the morning of the sixth day out of Cincinnati we entered a great harbor thronged with ocean shipping and clamorous with gulls, passed through miles of droning and friendly whistle-welcome, and tied up beside a vessel odorous with bags of coffee from Brazil.

We were in New Orleans, and Mardi Gras was just ahead.

CHAPTER V

BY CARE FORGOT

I WAS under a spell. I have never been quite free from it since, as a boy, I saw New Orleans, shared a room with my uncle in Rampart Street, ante-bellum habitat—though I knew it not—of free quadroon concubines, and every evening brought back a pail of oysters from the French Market, which the devout and sprightly little old Creole dame who ran the house stewed with strange herbs and served for us on the back porch. There was a show, she said, which we surely must see, for it was "jus' like Heaven." It was *The Black Crook!* I did not see it then, but I did attend a show in the old French Opera House, which went up in flames some twenty years ago, and there these eyes beheld the dashing Beauregard— that great general who might have matched Lee's career, had not Jefferson Davis, who rather fancied himself as a "strategist," judged him wrongly and meddled too much.

That visit was so long ago that streetcars were drawn by mules with bells tinkling at their throats and the warships in the river were wooden battlewagons; all the city cisterns were on platforms above ground, some of them ranged in three tiers atop of each other, and my recollection is that I drank only rain water. The Mint on Esplanade Street was still coining gold and silver. A statue of Henry Clay, since removed, stood on Canal Street in a posture of eloquence, and under it the pedestal on which Ben Butler had caused to be carved in 1862 the orator's most forthright antislavery utterance. In our bedroom was an odd little night lamp—a tumbler half full of water, a layer of olive oil over the water, and floating on the oil a cork with a tiny wick in it; it gave about as much light as a firefly.

We went to bed early, save for one night when my uncle took me to the Tivoli concert saloon on Royal Street. Entering, we sat down at a table, though I have since read that timid crowds of men contented themselves with standing upon the curbstone "to catch a glimpse of female limbs draped in gauze of pink and blue," limbs apt at dancing the cancan and the clodoche. Those that we saw were encased in black cotton tights, with just a handbreadth or so of skirt. Their wearers were robust young women of the whalebone epoch who sang from the stage and then came down and wandered from table to table, to my secret alarm.

Twenty years ago I saw New Orleans again and ever since I have wanted to return. No other city on earth has so held me.

The spell came upon me for a third time as I walked up from my boat to Canal Street and plunged into the Vieux Carré or French Quarter, on Royal Street, where its life beats highest. This is the old city, a compactly built district running only six blocks at right angles with the river and ten blocks roughly parallel with it. It should have been called the Latin Quarter, had not Paris preempted the name, for the original French Quarter with its wooden houses was destroyed by fire in 1788; a Spanish governor rebuilt it in brick faced with stucco, the Santo Domingo insurrections shortly thereafter peopled it with refugees, and later the fecund Italians moved in. The streets have haunting French names—Burgundy, Dauphine, Bourbon, Chartres, Iberville, Bienville, Conti, Esplanade—but the architecture is altogether Spanish, and two street signs suggest something more. One on the water front recites, "Furs, Alligator Skins and Pecans," and that is old-time American. Another, farther inland, reads, "Angelo

Glorioso, Winery," which is tops in Italian magniloquence.

Some French is spoken in the streets, but you seem most likely to hear it in the Toilettes des Messieurs. There is also an occasional bit of gallicized and antiquated English, such as this definite comment on crabs: "You not can cut dem de head off, for dat dey have not of head"—which I got out of Lafcadio Hearn. On the outer edges of the Quarter, where there are black and colored folk—New Orleans makes a distinction—you might hear snatches of Gombo, the quaint Negro Creole tongue.

Circumstances have molded New Orleans into the most interesting of American cities, with more in its history to win one's attention than in that of many countries. Its command of the mouth of the Mississippi established it in the seat of authority over the Republic's advance until the railroads came. Its oulook on the Gulf and the tropical islands that rim the Gulf made it a clearinghouse, and the last stronghold, of the privateers, smugglers, and buccaneers of the Spanish Main; made it a city of refuge for white families and their slave households driven by wars and black insurrections from the West Indies; made it also the home of ousted Latin-American rulers plotting counterrevolutions, and the starting point of filibustering adventures into Caribbean lands.

Strange as it seems, New Orleans was founded, and for a while ruled, by Canadians who came down the Great Lakes and the Mississippi. It shuttled back and forth among French, Spanish, and English overlords before the Americans took hold. Their coming brought another blood stream into an already cosmopolitan population, the so-called Kaintuck flatboatmen, whose rowdy ways outraged Creole sensibilities; a particular cause of offense being their reiterated assertions that they were of animal or reptilian descent—from "hosses, alligators, snappin' turtles."

Outstanding in the subsequent history of New Orleans were Jackson's victory over the British in 1815, which was the most important engagement in the War of 1812, and the capture of the city by Farragut's fleet in 1862, followed by the six-months' rule of Ben Butler, who may be called the first of American City Managers, nor yet the best. His order that all women who "insulted" Northern soldiers should be treated as women of the town caused Jefferson Davis to set a price on his head—"silly," says the Yankee historian Fiske, but "a not unnatural commentary," on Butler's conduct. Viewing the chicaneries and confiscations of his brief governorship in the light of recent events abroad, one might even call him the first of the Gauleiters. By contrast, the city holds in high regard Jean Lafitte, a pirate in the grand manner, whose rakish ships and cut-throat followers held Barataria Bay on the near-by Gulf coast, and whose gallantry at the Battle of New Orleans won words of praise from Jackson and an absolving proclamation from President Madison.

Stranger than its history is the location of the city. Its level is only a foot or so above the mean level of the Gulf, a hundred miles downstream. Water drains away from the Mississippi rather than toward it. You do not go down to the river, you go up to it. Even at low stages it stands a little above the street level. Wherefore, most of the burials are above ground, and the best architecture of New Orleans is in its white marble cemeteries. As a crowning singularity, the river flows north at Canal Street, the sun appearing to rise in the west.

In the same unusual category are the social history and outstanding customs of New Orleans. Best known of the latter is the series of balls and masquerades which begin in the winter holiday season and come to their climax, and close, with Mardi Gras; they have been held since colonial times and have been noteworthy since 1835. Dueling is no more, but in the decades just before the Civil War nearly every Creole of standing was at home with the rapier and sword cane, quick to resent even a fancied slight, and nearly as deadly in his bouts as a rattlesnake—that is, if he cared to be. The most famous duel was fought to avenge "the honor of the Mississippi" which a foreigner said was "a mere rill" compared to the rivers of Europe. With dueling went gambling, and after it came prizefighting; for years, when most states forbade such contests, New Orleans was the national capital of this vigorous sport.

As Flint has pointed out, Louisiana had the mildest slave code of any Southern state. Among other things, when the proportion of Negro blood in an individual had been diluted to one-thirty-second, he could no longer be held in bondage—a provision that anticipated the studies in evolution of Mendel, the Austrian monk. This, with the various manumissions by kindly slaveholders, brought a considerable free colored population into being—the quadroons, so-called. They never intermarried. The men married mulatto women. The quadroon women—many of them singularly beautiful, some of them educated in Europe—entered into domestic arrangements with white men; such arrangements were as near to marriage as law and custom would permit, and seemed to the women much the same thing. When their white partners married in their own race, the women were set up as proprietors of retail shops or as boardinghouse keepers. The social pacts which had this demure epilogue were negotiated at the celebrated quadroon balls, with the mothers of the girls attending as chaperons and business managers. While the Creole daughters wore white at their balls, the quadroons were garbed in vivid colors. Though their admission charges were double, these quadroon balls were the better attended. They have been called slave markets, but the term is too rough. There are now but few quadroons in New Orleans. If you believe its own writers, they have gone North and "gone white."

Concubinage is one thing, harlotry something else. It is said that the New Orleans brothels never had quadroon inmates. The history of the several segregated districts of the city has been written at large, and only two items will be entered here. At one house, which prided itself on its elegant hospitality, the mistress provided apples for the carriage horses which brought wealthy patrons to her door; and when they dressed the following morning they found that their clothes had been neatly pressed, their boots polished. The other item concerns a group of weeklies which in form, if not in spirit, anticipated modern tabloids, and were sold in cigar shops and saloons. Their "Society" columns contained such notes as this, "Madge Lester has returned from a trip and is back at Jessie Brown's," and this about somebody else, "Aside from the grandeur of her establishment, she has a score of beautiful women."

These matters are but memories now, and so is Congo Square where Negro slaves were allowed to dance on Sunday afternoons, and where, in the bamboula, cancan, calinda, and Congo, they wove their sense of barbaric rhythms into a wildly harmonious pattern. Voodoo worship, however, which is associated with this square, still has its followers, and amulets and magical powders command a market among Negroes and some of the whites.

Is this brief outline of New Orleans yesterdays too much a parade of gaieties, depravities, credulities? To balance the account a few statements at random: New Orleans is the second seaport of the country. Ninety steamship lines dock there. More distinguished men and women have lived in the narrow limits of the French Quarter than in any similar area, among its homes being those of Adelina Patti, Audubon, Gottschalk, Beauregard, Lafcadio Hearn, Judah P. Benjamin, Paul Morphy, John Slidell, Charles Gayarré, several governors, several ex-Presidents of Latin-American countries. In George W. Cable it had an interpreter of whom any city might be proud. It has a devout church-going population.

In the Vieux Carré I spent the better part of four days, eating there, shopping in a small way on that bewildering Royal Street, exploring one block after another, emerging when some colorful pageant passed by on flanking Canal Street, returning rather late at night to the dark, peaceful quiet of our steamboat, down among the coffee and banana ships. There, as on a floating hotel, I slept and had breakfast.

With friends from the boat I made a few excursions outside the Quarter: to the so-called Garden district, where white-columned houses stand amid palms and have lawns and fountains and blooming flowers all the year around; along Bayou St. John to the blue, crystal expanse of Lake Pontchartrain, which is only four miles from the river and is the city's back way to the Gulf; to the beautiful cemeteries which in very truth are cities of the dead, their streets lined with white marble chapels; to Congo Square where once the slaves congregated for voodoo dances.

But this narrative goes back, as its author did, to the French Quarter, stopping at only one place outside it; and St. Louis Cemetery is very near it. A brick wall surrounds an ancient graveyard, and in its crevices grasses have taken root. In places the wall is itself a mausoleum, with openings into which coffins are thrust—like long loaves of French bread in an outdoor oven—and then sealed. The wall incloses the strangest, the most haunting spot I know. Among banana trees, blooming rose bushes, and date palms heavy with purple fruit are the silent homes, marble and brick and stone, of men and women who walked the streets of New Orleans when the Republic was young. Their habitations, all above ground, have doors, windows, and little balconies with wrought-iron grilles, even as those in the near-by Quarter.

After I was there twenty years ago—a pilgrimage that took me, coming and going, through streets where women called from the windows; Storeyville it used to be called —I wrote some verses based on the lovely Creole names on the headstones, all of those cited being of women. This time, to be fair, I noted not only Julie, Marie, Celestine, Florestine, and Mathilde, but also Hippolyte, Armand, Alcide, Alexandre, Lucien, Auguste. I beg leave to print the verses written aforetime.

I had a dream of women fair
Within a crumbling close,
Between the ranks of cedars where
Their names the marble chapels bear,
And droops and dreams the rose:
Once more the earth knew Honorine,
Babette and Heloise,
And wore the mirth of Jacqueline,
Zabette, Nichette, Denyse.

The morning filled the Place of Arms,
And church bells clanged above
The steel that spoke of war's alarms,

The silks arraying youthful charms,
The young hearts prone to love;
And fleet the smiles of Honorine,
Babette and Heloise,
But sweet the wiles of Jacqueline,
Zabette, Nichette, Denyse.

Along the river bank at night,
They moved, a merry throng
Of Creole dandies apt for fight
And Creole maids with eyes alight
And lips that framed a song:
I played the lute for Honorine,
Babette and Heloise,
And paid my suit to Jacqueline,
Zabette, Nichette, Denyse . . .

By certain shuttered streets they pass
Who leave the burial ground;
And there I saw a pleasant lass,
Of such as spend no time at mass,
But I looked not around:
For I was knight to Honorine,
Babette and Heloise,
And I had plight with Jacqueline,
Zabette, Nichette, Denyse!

In the Quarter I saw the things that everybody seeks out
—Pirates' Alley; the old Absinthe House and other haunts
of Lafitte, in which the *Buccaneer* film had awakened new
interest; the "dead church" of St. Anthony, the home of
Adelina Patti, the Café des Refugées, the site of the St.
Louis Hotel where Galsworthy saw a white horse ambling
through deserted courts, the Gate of the Lions, the Court

of the Two Sisters, the Spanish Courtyard, the Old Sazerac House, the Cornstalk Fence, the Courtyard of the Vine, the Patio Royal, the Haunted House of Mme. Lalaurier whose cruelties to her slaves incited—so the story runs—a mild insurrection of townsmen; the Cabildo, once the Spanish parliament building, now a museum; the old St. Louis Cathedral, commanding the Place d'Armes on the river front; the statue of Jackson, whose name the square now bears; the imposing apartment buildings erected on two sides of the square a century ago by Baroness Fontalba, and just beyond, the French Market with its fish, fruits, and coffee stands.

Of course, I dined at Antoine's and other eating places of the Quarter, and there discussed such matters as gumbo Creole, and bisque écrevisse, and frog legs, and red snapper and pompano en papelotte, and shrimp remoulade, and Bayou Cook oysters on the half shell—which go very well with beer. I brought a pearly half shell away for an ash tray. At a number of cocktail lounges one could dance in the late afternoon, and a notably smooth concoction was the Sazerac. The Ramos gin fizz also had a legendary appeal.

Some of the handsome old residences with their courtyards, gilded mirror frames and black marble mantelpieces —that of General Beauregard was outstanding—we were permitted to enter. But the only interior I note here is the Convent of the Holy Family on Orleans Street, an order of Negro nuns. Sister Conception, country-bred and slightly French, met me and a friend at the door, and drew the color line at once, turning a group of Negro callers who arrived at the same time over to another nun. The convent was once the Orleans Theatre, where the free quadroon women of the city—by all accounts the world's most beautiful— gave their famous dances, and only young white men, the elite of the town, danced with them. I saw the ballroom floor, and the open court where amorous couples sipped wine and ices under the stars, and the inscription which the Sisters have placed above the stairway, "I have chosen rather to be an abject in the house of the Lord than to dwell in the temple with the sinners." With a sweet tolerance the nun spoke of these things. In the mellow-hued chapel upstairs, she told us how a leaden image of St. Jean (if I get his name right) extinguished a threatening fire downstairs when thrown into it.

At some time I must have been too near a slot machine, for my change pocket held many nickels, each of which, as it dropped into the poor box—so Sister Conception declared —meant another meal for an orphan.

What makes the French Quarter distinctive is that, first of all, its yards and gardens are hidden from the street. A blank wall awakens expectation and surmise, turns the prose of a dwelling into verse, into blank verse, if you please—unless you surmise a plashing fountain, and then thought becomes lyrical. The fountain will be in a court, or patio, with double galleries looking down upon it, and outside staircases connecting them; and a canary singing on the upper gallery, or perhaps a green popinjay, harsh of voice. In the court—I had luncheon in such a place—are palms and banana plants and fig trees; grass, perhaps, or perhaps a tiled or sanded pavement, the blue sky overhead.

Exteriors are in limewashes of tinted stucco: cream, mustard yellow, pink, green, slate-blue, sometimes red. All houses have green shutters before windows and even before doors, which are deeply recessed. An unpainted wooden stoop with elbows for sitters leads to the street. Along the basements are small, grated cellar windows like flattened portholes. The passageway beside the house seems to be its main entrance; on the jealous boards which shut it off from the street are the house number, mailbox and doorbell. Along the second floor is an overhanging balcony with iron grillwork. Under each window of the third floor, if there is one, are small individual balconies, also with grillwork.

In these grilles is much of the magic of the Quarter. Older houses have wrought-iron balconies, made in Seville or hand-hammered by slaves in forges at home. The newer houses have cast-iron work. These grilles give the streets an atmosphere of play and fantasy. I saw a monkey climbing along one—a feat not to be copied by humans, for here and there sharp, cruel claws of iron make the adventures of porch climbers and second-storv workers something to be sorry for.

It was interesting to figure out patterns woven into this iron lace. Favorite motive was the oak leaf and acorn; next, perhaps grape leaves and grape clusters. Other designs that I observed were passionflowers, fleur de lys, morning glories, harps, lyres, crossed cannon, cupids, crossed arrows, daggers, doves, conventionalized trees, lodge emblems, monograms.

I saw four of the pageants of the pre-Lenten season: the children's carnival of Nor, the krewe of Proteus, the parade of Rex, and the procession of the king of the Zulus—this last a coconut-tossing African revel with a touch of humorous satire in it. The celebrants rode in gorgeous symbolical floats, wore rather simpering, good-natured masks, and tossed jewelry and other trinkets into outstretched hands. But for these maskers there would be no carnival, yet the crowd itself, glutting a thoroughfare one hundred and eighty feet wide, was the real thing. As the crowd passed, I made brief notes and here is the verbatim record:

Pirates, pierettes, punchinellos, gypsies, men in nightgowns, men in brassieres, imitation Africans, cowled

monks, Scotch Highlanders, cannibals with naked bodies
and horned heads, harem beauties, female Uncle Sams, un-
convincing lady ruffians, those phallic hand balloons, bare
female legs, bullfighters, waitresses, silken-trousered sing-
song girls, other trousered dames, geishas, Balkanesses, girl
cowboys, jockeys, courtiers and caballeros, the Grim Reaper
and his scythe, a turbaned Turk, skeleton and death's head,
as I live two goons from the *Times-Star* comic strip, gilt-
armored crusaders, crinoline misses, more bare legs, ging-
ham girls, brows bandanna-bound, madras tignons, "Hello,
Big Boy" (wotta girl!), more legs, togas, candystick trousers, dunce caps, overalls, slacks, shorts, legs.

Men and women were dancing in the streets and in saloons on the lower end of Canal Street as I walked back to
the boat to change for the Rex Ball, with which Mardi
Gras closes. At this high-lighted function I found a multitude in formal attire, a floor of beguiling smoothness, dance
strains insinuating and adept. Parading before the royal
court with a partner from our boat, I had a near view of
Rex and his pretty queen. Wearing the traditional false
whiskers of his role, he looked quite like the King of
Hearts. Tall though she is, when the queen smiled, I was
minded of Sonja Henie. I played hard for that smile, and
giving myself every benefit of doubt, boasted afterward
that it had been vouchsafed.

On the stroke of midnight, revels ended and Lent came
in. An hour later our boat was on its way upstream.

CHAPTER VI

RED BOUNDARY LINE

OF THAT Red River—there are several—which is one of the Mississippi's three big western daughters, I have seen only the mouth. We passed it on our journey to and from New Orleans, midway between Natchez and Baton Rouge, on an old boundary line, the thirty-second degree of latitude, between Spain and the United States. Yet my personal acquaintance with it goes a little farther, for I have had a glimpse of the Atchafalaya and more than a glimpse of Bayou Teche; the former is a bayou by which the Red sends part of its burden to the Gulf, the latter was once the lower course of that stream.

Red River has more to tell that is significant or strange than all but one or two of the waterways of the continent, and most of its story seems to be nearly forgotten. Part of that story it shares with the Arkansas and Missouri. Ascending these three by pirogue, keelboat, and steamboat, men found themselves on a vaster frontier than that of the Old West. The Great American Forest with its humid depths and its shadows where painted savages lurked, was left behind, and in its stead were rolling prairies, high plains, lands of little rain—an almost continental area which in the older school geographies was called the Great American Desert. As on the earlier frontier, there were savages and buffaloes; but the savages were plains tribes mounted on small horses stolen from the Mexican settlements, and the buffaloes were in great herds which followed the sun in search of pasture, instead of straitened columns moving from salt lick to salt lick.

Men in this Farther West lived, not in log cabins, but in covered wagons, canvas tents, skin lodges, sod houses, squat adobe dwellings that were rude copies of a spacious Spanish style. Their quest at first was for adventurous living and for gold, rather than for homesteads. Government forts, held by troops of cavalry, went with them or ahead of them, and this had not been the rule before, at least in Kentucky and Tennessee. The new country was dotted with clumps of buffalo grass, with mesquite bushes and sage brush, monumented with cactus columns, populous with prairie-dog towns. There were rivers flowing only at night, which were thought to follow the moon and have tides like the sea. Eagerly sought water holes, and wet-weather ponds that had been buffalo wallows, were scattered over the plains. On a distant horizon was the loom of snowy, dreamlike mountains with the promise of gold to lure men toward the sunset.

When they went into this western world by the Red River, they came upon a singular barrier. In histories and travel narratives this is the Raft, printed in capital letters as one might speak of the Gulf or the Desert, and commonly dismissed without description. But it did not float. It was more like a roof, or a bridge, perhaps a covered bridge; the river crept under it or coursed around it. Save for its size, it might have been called a permanent log jam. It was an accumulation of logs, stumps, whole trees, and miscellaneous drift, which extended from bank to bank— and in some places that was several miles.

Freshets and its own decay had given the raft a thin, rich soil on which broomstraw, bushes, and small willows were growing. Usually one could walk across it without wetting the feet. A New Orleans savant, who compares it to an old, worn-out field that had been abandoned to grow up again, gives its length as about one hundred and thirty miles. An-

other writer reports that in 1832 it extended from Loggy
Bayou to Carolina Bluffs, a distance of one hundred and
sixty-five miles. Farther up the river, beyond Shreveport,
was another raft thirty-two miles long; but these figures
overlap. There was a third and shorter raft on the Atchafalaya.

When white men first set eyes on the Red River raft, it
may have been four hundred years old. It is thought that
at some remote time the Mississippi was high and the Red
low, and the bigger river backed into its affluent, creating
still water at the latter's mouth; drift which came down
Red, instead of passing out when the Mississippi fell,
spread from bank to bank, anchored itself there to channel snags, and tangled up into an impregnable barrier.
Everything which descended later was held fast and built
into the structure, the raft extending itself upstream perhaps a mile and a half a year. Its lower and older reaches
rotted, broke off and floated away after about four years,
leaving open water beyond; but this disintegration was
only at half the rate of accretions from above.

Thus the raft, although stationary, moved upstream and
steadily grew longer. It had backed off nearly four hundred
miles from the river's mouth before the government grappled with it. When Alexandria and Natchitoches were first
settled, even then the raft was behind them. It has wrought
permanent changes in the topography of the region, divert-
ing the river's flow into lateral bayous and transforming
prairies into lakes. Early boatmen and even small steamboats turned into these bayous, regaining the main channel
days afterward in their ascent into the interior.

In 1833, army engineers under Captain Henry M. Shreve
tackled the raft. He had a so-called snag-eradicator and two
tenders. The snagger was a double steamboat, the bows
connected with a stout beam plated with iron. Under a

heavy head of steam the boat would ram a snag, which
would break off at the bottom and drift away. Decaying
lower portions of the raft yielded to less strenuous measures and were easily grappled off. Thus in the first season a
hundred miles were pulled to pieces and floated down river.
Navigation was opened as far up as Coates Bluff which,
then uninhabited, is now Shreveport, near the western
boundary of Louisiana, with a population of about a hundred thousand, the state's second largest city. It took five
years to complete the task and enable boats to pass from
the lower to the upper river. More than once since that
time, the raft has reappeared.

Far above the Great Raft, the Red River flowed through
another barrier, of living trees, not dead ones, which let
the waterway alone, but against land travel interposed
something half hedge and half wall. In older travel narratives this was known as Cross Timbers. It extended from
the Brazos for four hundred miles across the plains to the
Arkansas and varied in width from five to thirty miles.
Josiah Gregg, who saw it in 1833, calls it the fringe of the
great prairies. East of it were verdurous lands, west of it
was semidesert, and it almost cut off communication between the two. The timber was dwarfish and choked with
underbrush such as blackjacks, post oaks, shin oaks. Stunted
by continued inroads from what were called the burning
prairies, vegetation sprang up anew and in spots became
so matted with greenbriars and wild grapevines as to form
almost impenetrable roughs—hiding places for wild beasts
and wild men.

Captain Marcy, who led an expedition up Red River in
1852, and found Cross Timbers so crowded with trees that
wagons could scarcely get between them, has a striking passage in his report: "This forms a boundary line, dividing
the country suited to agriculture from the great prairies,

which, for the most part, are arid and destitute of timber. It seems to have been designed as a natural barrier between civilized man and the savage." On one side was good farm land and tall timber with plenty of water. "On the other side commence those barren and desolate wastes, where but few small streams greet the eye of the traveller, and these are soon swallowed up by the thirsty sands. From the point where Red River leaves the timbered lands, the entire face of the country changes its character."

Of course those thickets are no more, but the regions which they bound are as they were.

Marcy found the source of the Red River—Long had sought it in vain in 1809—in another region which lies just west of Cross Timbers. It bore a haunting name. This was known as Llano Estacado or Staked Plain, allegedly because the Mexicans had marked with stakes a way across its empty spaces; but may not the so-called stakes have been cactus pillars set there by the Lord? On the eastern edge of this plateau, as Marcy reports, the south or principal fork of Red River was half a mile wide, flowing over a sandy bed with but little water in it and flanked by hills and gullies impassable to wagons. With a dozen horsemen he climbed the heights and kept on up the bed of the river.

He found himself in a valley with precipitous walls, and the river only a hundred feet wide. Farther up it contracted to twenty feet. The stone escarpments rose to a height of eight hundred feet, gradually closed in, and finally united above a long, narrow corridor where there was perpetual twilight. From the canyon a spring flashed down the rocks, and that was the source of Red River. Noble were its beginnings, framed in what appeared to be castle walls.

Llano Estacado, where the Red rises, is the Balcony of Texas. Though on the map it does not loom importantly in the vast Texas spaces, it has an area of thirty thousand square miles, is larger than ten states of the Union. It was long a land of legend, and to be shunned. Mexican herders and Indians told Gregg that it was waterless during nine months of the year, that most of its few perennial streams were too brackish to drink from, and that some of the water holes on the only safe route in the dry season were fifty or more miles apart and hard to find.

"This most inhospitable and dreaded salt desert," is the picture the Indians left with the white explorer. Other travelers spoke of the shimmering cheats of the mirage. A more realistic—and quite recent—account is in the recollections of Lane, veteran army scout, who says that in the 1870's the Red River's canyon source was a camping place for savage tribes; that the plateau had been stripped of its timber by Indian fires, and that then "white men brought in too many cattle and ate out the Staked Plain." At the springs of Red a number of plains tribes had surrendered to General Mackenzie.

In a theater where all seats are free or all held at equal price, and where the balcony is reached by steep flights of stairs, the ground floor fills up first, and unless there is a crowd the balcony may remain almost unoccupied. That is a parable of the Staked Plain. On the eastern side its walls rise precipitously and white limestone cap rock rims them. From nearly two thousand feet above, it looks down on the rest of Texas. Atop, it is a vast level plain which extends from the one hundredth meridian to and beyond the eastern border of New Mexico, and from the Texas Panhandle south to the latitude of New Mexico's lower border. On his earlier expedition to Santa Fe, Marcy abandoned the Staked Plain completely to the prairie dogs and the owl and rattlesnake tenants of their towns: "It is a region almost as vast and trackless as the ocean—a land where no man, either savage or civilized, permanently abides."

Events have made a mockery of this somber picture. The Staked Plain is now a land of windmills and water, of white farmhouses and white cotton fields. It produces more cotton than South Carolina. The northern part of the plateau is the largest wheat-producing area of Texas. All this has come to pass since the end of the World War. The collapse of 1920 ruined the big ranchers of the South Plain—as the lower part of Llano Estacado is called; their land was to be had for a song, and young farmers and their families moved in. From fifty to three hundred feet below the surface there was found an inexhaustible supply of pure water. The plain is high enough to raise wheat, too high for the boll weevil pest, not adapted for corn but friendly to the grain sorghums, and its cattle and hogs can remain all year in the open.

The one hundredth meridian, which bounds the plateau to the east, has been from the beginning of the Republic a boundary both in popular tradition and in treaties of sovereign lands in which Red River has played a part. The meridian was long thought to be the dead line for rainfall, nature's own barrier between the desert and the sown. Meridian and river, together with two other waterways and the country's greatest mountain range, drew the boundaries of the young Republic with Spain, and with Mexico when it became Spain's successor.

By the treaty with Spain in 1819, the boundary between this country and the province of New Spain ran from the Gulf of Mexico north along the Sabine River and across country to Red, west along Red to the meridian, north along this to the Arkansas, and thence northwest along the latter to the Rockies, which it followed to British Columbia. The boundary was not far from three thousand miles long, half of it formed by the three rivers. More than five hundred miles of it followed the meanderings of Red, its tinted tide repeating the hue with which boundaries are delineated on maps.

Although the romance that is in all borders suggests itself at a glance, this rambling international boundary would be little remembered were it not the boundary between Louisiana and Texas and on two sides between Texas and Oklahoma. Except its pink water, Red River seems to owe everything it has to the courts rather than to the Lord.

These decreed that the south branch was the main river; that the south bank of the branch was the old international boundary determined in the treaty with Spain; that the river valley had not changed, as claimed by Oklahoma, since 1819; that inside the valley the banks have been altered by accretion rather than island-building as claimed by the nation; and that, in fine, the boundary between Texas and Oklahoma ran along that place on the south side of the south branch of Red where the cut-bank (where vegetation ceased) met the sand flat, which latter belonged to the nation. Oklahoma's claim that the river had moved north and was holding stolen land in and beyond its wide valley was nonsuited.

Explanation of this grapple between states, involving sovereignty over what seemed to be worthless sand bars covered by every rise of Red River, is that oil was discovered in the valley in 1919, a pool of great richness underlying the river itself near the (always significant) one hundredth meridian.

Oklahoma recently lost again, in the Supreme Court this time, in a controversy with the Federal Government which it charged with violating state rights by projecting a power dam at Denison on the Texas boundary—again near the hundredth meridian—under pretense of flood control.

Perhaps the most singular expedition of the Civil War was that both by land and water—the latter a dozen iron-clads under Porter—up Red River in 1864 to seize Shreveport, then capital of Louisiana. It had rather the odor of a cotton speculation and little has been said about it since. The Federal commander Banks, who conducted it, did so under protest. Ambushed and defeated at the Battle of Sabine Forks by Dick Taylor, who had eleven thousand men to his thirty-one thousand, he withdrew to Alexandria. There began a retreat, which redeemed in some measure what had gone before.

The river was falling. It was feared that low water would trap all of Porter's squadron, comprising some of the best ironclads of the North's Mississippi fleet; that they would have to be blown up to prevent their capture; and that thus the South might regain for a time command of the Mississippi. But the ingenuity of a Michigan lumberman, familiar with splash dams, constrained the Southern river to do the North's bidding. "If damning would get the fleet over," scoffed the incredulous Porter, "it would have been afloat long before." But damming did the trick. The baffled army, under direction of Lumberman Bailey, came to the rescue of the stranded fleet.

At Alexandria were rapids a mile long filled with rocks, through which the river, some seven hundred feet wide and from four to six feet deep, was running at ten miles an hour. Bailey undertook to make what he called a tree-dam to raise its level. Three thousand soldiers with a thousand horses, mules, and oxen and two hundred army wagons toiled night and day upon it. Oaks, elms, and pines for cribbing were felled, stripped of their branches and dragged to the north bank, while flatboats brought in stone. On the south bank, where there was no timber, old mills, barns, and sugar houses were torn down, cribs were made of the lumber, and bricks from chimneys, stones from foundations, and iron railroad tracks were used to sink them. At the end of the dams on both banks four large coal barges filled with stone and brick were sunk. This left a chute seventy-six feet wide. Supplementary wing dams were built above after two of the coal barges were swept away.

Convinced that the fleet was doomed, and entertained by songs from the Union camp, Confederate troops watched from a distance. The sequel was not to their liking. Back of the dams the river rose more than six feet and through the chute the gunboats dashed to safety in the open river below. It had taken the army only a dozen days to build the dam; it would have taken a private contractor a year, said the Secretary of the Navy. The skeptical Porter acclaimed it as "the best engineering feat ever performed," and he and his officers presented Bailey with a sword and a purse of three thousand dollars.

Perhaps Bailey had remembered the Great Raft.

Here may be taken up the story of Red River navigation, which for a long time was all below the Raft.

The best descriptions of Red River—still very much as it used to be—are those of the early explorers. They made only one important error, guessing its length as twenty-five hundred miles instead of thirteen hundred. Along the upper river they noted the characteristic details of arid America: brackish water, salines, quicksands, stunted brush, tumbleweed, dry creek beds that were practicable highways for men and horses; other creeks bordered with pecan trees, black walnuts, elms, hackberries, cottonwoods, wild China trees, willows; here and there an Indian village with lodges like haystacks, and about them cornfields and thrifty patches of pumpkins, melons, and beans.

Marcy's account gives the clearest picture. Below the Staked Plain he found the river "a broad, shallow stream, six hundred and fifty yards wide, running over a bed of sand." From this point, he adds, "it flows through an arid prairie country almost entirely destitute of trees, over a broad bed of light and shifting sands, for a distance, measured upon its sinuosities, of some five hundred miles . . . It then enters a country covered with forest trees of gigantic dimensions, growing upon an alluvial soil of the most pre-eminent fertility. Below the Great Raft a chain of lakes continues to skirt the river for more than a hundred miles. These lakes are filled and emptied alternately as the floods in Red River rise and fall; they serve as reservoirs, which in the inundations receive a great quantity of water and as the flood subsides empty their contents gradually."

The French of Louisiana began the navigation of the Red River very early, sending an expedition up it in 1714 to form a settlement at Natchitoches. In 1730 they sent another to drive the Natchez Indians from the Red and Black River districts, capturing and selling a number as slaves to Santo Domingo. In 1749 the province of Natchitoches had sixty whites and two hundred Negroes, and raised cattle, corn, rice, and tobacco. By the end of the century, Natchitoches had a population of eight hundred.

With the Louisiana Purchase in 1803, American exploration and settlement began, the first travel being in keelboats of from ten to fifty tons. The first steamboat on the river went up to Alexandria in 1820. By 1825 there were seven packets running to Natchitoches and making thirty-six voyages a year. In 1831 removal of the Choctaws to Indian Territory began, mainly by way of the Arkansas,

but also up the Red and the tributary Ouachita and thence
overland. The Raft was destroyed because it cut off navigation between the upper and lower river, hampering the
removal of the Civilized Indians and also the movement
of troops and supplies to the new forts set up to protect
them from their wild plains kinsmen.

Thereafter steamboats multiplied, mostly small craft of
around a hundred tons and drawing less than twenty inches.
About seventy-five of them were on the river between 1835
and 1840. Perhaps twoscore were stationed above and below
Shreveport in the Civil War, including a number of Confederate rams, gunboats, and ironclads. After the war the
New Orleans and Red River Transportation Company had
nine boats running. Its last boat made its last trip up Red
River in 1882—perhaps a significant date in what has been
called the pageant of the packets; the railroads were now
everywhere in the Western country.

In 1880 the imports on Red River above the mouth of
Black were valued at nearly thirteen million dollars; by
1923 river commerce had dwindled to four hundred and
sixty thousand, largely down-bound rafted logs. There is
present navigation as far as Alexandria, about one hundred
and forty miles up. Most of the towboats and barges which
enter Red River, however, turn off after thirty-five miles
and go north on the Ouachita-Black River (one river with
two names) which is six hundred miles long, has locks and
dams, and is navigable to Camden, Arkansas, a distance of
three hundred and fifty miles. Forty-nine steamboats with
their barges were on that river in 1938, carrying fish, logs,
sugar, molasses, cotton, beans, dried fruit, fertilizer, and
gasoline.

Cramer called Red River in 1814 the American Nile, its
lower valley perhaps the richest in the world. Flint who
knew it well, and for a time lived beside it, may have had

the same thought in 1824 when he likened it to "a serpentine and very deep canal," and spoke of the snake-haunted cypress swamps that flanked it and the shoals of alligators on its sand bars. On modern maps it never quite reaches the Mississippi, though this is merely a matter of nomenclature. Four miles above its mouth the Atchafalaya takes off from it and follows its former channel to the Gulf. What of Red reaches the Mississippi from that point is called Old River. When we passed the mouth on our New Orleans expedition it seemed about the size of the Tennessee, though with its caving banks it looked more like a lesser Mississippi. Flint speaks of its "bloody water." However, it was high when we saw it and a chocolate-brown.

CHAPTER VII

THE TRAIL OF TEARS

FOR days on the way up the Mississippi after Mardi Gras ended we buffeted the flood waters of the Arkansas, which moved upon it. They carried a message from far-off places that I knew. I had heard their low thunder in the Royal Gorge of Colorado. One of the river's many fountains I had seen when I crossed the Continental Divide and the state line of New Mexico. This was at Raton Pass, seventy-six hundred feet in air. As the train descended, I had a glimpse of the twin Spanish Peaks —distant snowy battlements that mingled with the clouds but were no part of them. Below was the town of Trinidad and a stream called Purgatory which pays a scanty toll to the Arkansas at La Junta. Thereafter I followed the main river for hours across the high plains of Colorado. It was not like the streams from which I had come in the arid Southland, and which—with their vertical banks, flat floors, and a dampness in them that was little more than morning dew—were easy to mistake for sunken highways. The Arkansas was an indubitable river, and had water and bordering willows.

Though little is heard about it except in the June floods, it is one of the great rivers of the country. Of all the tributaries of the Mississippi none starts so high in air, and, save the Missouri, none travels so far. It is fourteen hundred and sixty miles long. Small steamboats have gone up to the Kansas town of Wichita—six hundred and fifty miles. Rising in the same part of Colorado out of which flow the Rio Grande, the Platte, and the Colorado, it traverses a

88

corner of Kansas and the States of Oklahoma and Arkansas, dropping nearly two miles in its journey to the Mississippi. In places it is a mile wide. Bent's Fort, finest trading post of the West, was in a wide curve of the upper river. Far below, Coronado crossed it in his quest of Quivira. Forty miles from its mouth is Arkansas Post, established in 1686, oldest permanent settlement in the Mississippi Valley, once a famed trading center for Indian peltries, later the territorial capital. Just above its mouth were the legendary silver mines of John Law's dreams, and there he erected his short-lived duchy. At its mouth the body of De Soto, discoverer of the Mississippi, was sunk in a weighted log in 1542.

The best early accounts of the Arkansas are by John Bradbury, who was on it in 1810, and Nuttall, who went up from Arkansas Post to Fort Smith in 1819 in what he called a large shell. Both noted the redness of the water. Nuttall found a decadent French population at the post. From Indians he obtained honey in a deerskin bottle. He saw vast tracts of cane along the river bends, and was told there were panthers in the woods behind them. Once he came upon a herd of bison. Between the Arkansas and the Red he traversed "extensive woodless plains where no echo answers the voice, and its tones die away in boundless and enfeebled undulations."

Perhaps the most recent account of a trip upon it was jotted down in Thanksgiving week of 1920, in a journal to which I have had access. Its author, a friend of mine, took the trip as guest of the steamboat *Ralph Hicks*, which was towing a laden barge to Pine Bluff, the first direct shipment by water from St. Louis in more than thirty years.

On a late afternoon his steamboat swung into the Arkansas, passing the site of the drowned county seat of Napoleon which, says the diarist, "I did not see, for nobody knows where it is." It took half an hour of pushing, sounding, and backing before the boat could get into the river. In another half hour it tied up for the night against Big Island, which is formed by the Mississippi, White, and Arkansas rivers and the Arkansas River cut-off. Some house-boat families lived there among their goats. The following morning the narrator was amazed to find the river narrow and tortuous, with a swift current of extremely red water, much of it discharging into the Mississippi through the cut-off over to White River. When the boat came to a rail-road drawbridge—"the first thing I had seen, of earth, tim-ber or iron, that looked half-way permanent"—the pilot scanned the channel, decided it was no longer under the drawspan, and ducked under the permanent span.

Beyond the cut-off, the Arkansas widened and deepened, and travel was better. The voyagers found two daymarks, "the only aids to navigation on the river," and both had become hindrances. "I was told all day," notes the narra-tor, "that we would lie for the night at Arkansas Post, first capital of Arkansas; but when we got there I saw, as usual, nothing." With the boat's master he set out on a moon-light walk to the post. They threaded a cotton field, fol-lowed a hog path for more than a mile—and found the old bed of the river, still half full of water, lying across their way. Just beyond it but out of reach were a general store and post office, about all that was left of the ancient town.

The third day was Thanksgiving, and the midday meal aboard was "terrible"—no potatoes, a wild duck too nearly raw to eat, nothing on the table but canned soup, canned peaches, and prunes. However, in the afternoon an officer shot two wild ducks, and himself cooked and served them smoking hot for supper. Meanwhile, they passed the first Southern plantation home they had seen, though now and then over the levees they glimpsed the roofs of farmhouses

and barns. They bivouacked at Greenback Plantation. On
the fourth day they found a crowd of spectators awaiting
them as they approached Pine Bluff. Having shot a wild
goose, they sat down to a farewell dinner before going
ashore.

Ten years before, Captain Sam G. Smith, coeditor of the
Waterways Journal, was on the Arkansas as master of the
packet *Grant* which went up as far as Fort Smith and also
ran excursions from Little Rock. Above the latter, he tells
me that the Arkansas is the most beautiful of rivers, with
gravel bottom, a framework of towering bluffs, and here
and there singular pinnacles rising from the plain to a
height of nearly five hundred feet.

For the first half of every year there is a four-foot channel from the Missisippi at least as far as up to Pine Bluff;
for the second half, a two-foot channel. Periodic floods raise
the lower river as much as sixty feet. Two snagboats toil at
an endless task set by the caving banks and a shifting channel. One year recently the boats removed fourteen hundred
snags and felled hundreds of trees on the sliding shores.
There is a modest traffic—no passengers at all in 1938, but
a score of steamers, and twelve hundred barges which carried sand, gravel, wood, paper, and logs—the total value of
cargoes being a little less than three hundred thousand
dollars.

The era of steamboating on the inland rivers began in
1817 when Henry Shreve's *Washington*, the first boat that
traveled on the water instead of in it, went down the Ohio
and Mississippi. Three years afterward, according to one
account, there were ten packets on the Arkansas. I have
the names of forty that were upon it a score of years later.
Actually, they were numbered by hundreds.

Both Federal and Confederate gunboats patrolled the

Arkansas in the Civil War. They met at the battle of
Arkansas Post in January, 1863, in the operations that
preluded the siege of Vicksburg. Wishing to redeem the
frustration of his Yazoo River campaign and give his idle
troops something to do, Sherman suggested an attack on
the post to his superior, McClernand, who undertook it in
person with Porter leading a flotilla of Union gunboats.
The post was a four-bastioned fort on a bend of the Arkansas with earthworks running from the river to an impassable bayou. Five thousand Confederates defended it. After
some resistance they surrendered and their six gunboats
were burned.

Before that engagement, the river shared in three great
chapters of American history. Afterward, nothing much
happened, the decline in steamboating setting in there as
elsewhere. Though the Arkansas is classed as navigable to
the mouth of the Neosho in Oklahoma four hundred and
sixty miles above its own mouth, it now has no commercial
navigation save in the eighty-mile reach from Pine Bluff
down. Above that point, the government concluded in
1928 that channel depths were too uncertain for further
effort. Below it, constant snagging keeps the waterway open.

The first and most significant of three services performed
by the river was the removal of the Five Civilized Tribes
into the West. A century ago the Arkansas was the only
highway from the Mississippi to the Indian Territory, from
the settled lands of the whites to plains with no inhabitants
save roving bands of red buffalo hunters. To reach the
mouth of the Arkansas and there begin the last stage of
their journey, the tribes went by land and water—down the
Tennessee, Ohio, and Mississippi; across Florida to Tampa
Bay, down the Alabama to Mobile Bay; from either port
by steamship to New Orleans, and thence by steamboat up

river to the Arkansas. Some parties made the whole journey overland, traversing Kentucky, Illinois, and Missouri on ponies or in oxcarts.

Not all of them left. Some years ago I spent a few days among the Eastern Band of Cherokees in the mountain fastnesses of North Carolina. They were descendants of men who a century ago had resolved to die rather than be taken West. The army officer whose task it was to get them out, a humane realist, did not want to see his men killed while pursuing an invisible foe down impossible ravines and over impassable peaks in the Land of the Sky. Constituting himself at once President and Senate, he entered into some sort of unofficial treaty which permitted the band to remain; he got by with it, and there they are.

I lived in the house of a Cherokee in the Great Smokies and called on many of his people. They were kindly in the grave aboriginal way. Since then I have been keenly interested in their nation. Its members are the most numerous, most industrious, and most civilized of Indian peoples and, thanks to Sequoyah and his syllabary, almost as literate as the whites. They play baseball, they seem to like work, and they are at home in the prize ring—all of these things minor confirmations perhaps of my notion that a long vista of civilized life is behind them; that they were the mound builders.

They are a proud people. Into my office one day not long ago came two vivid young women, a brunette and a redhead, whom I had met in the Dakota Black Hills. Before we went out to a restaurant the brunette dug a small, vicious-looking automatic from her handbag and placed it in a drawer of my desk. It was a useful companion, of course, for two damsels crossing the continent alone in a car, but its owner handled it with a casual assurance that took me aback. "Did I never tell you," she said, "that I am a Cherokee? When I was a girl in Oklahoma it used to grieve me that I was not a full blood. It's all right now."

She was the descendant of a people living in the South whom Andrew Jackson and men like him called "wandering savages," "children of the forest," and "savage hunters," but who in fact were a nation of farmers, merchants, innkeepers, and artisans, who sent their corn, cattle, cotton, and fabrics down all the navigable rivers to New Orleans. Their first forty years under the flag show up well enough beside the first forty years of Puritan New England, and they had wrought for themselves a more enlightened government.

The major part of the Cherokees went on with the sixty thousand Indians who left the land of their fathers between 1830 and 1843 and journeyed toward the setting sun. Their route westward is known as The Trail of Tears.

Of the army officers who executed President Jackson's removal program, it is to be said that, except in the Seminole Wars, they discharged with humanity duties which many of them detested. The case against Jackson is that he evaded the pledges of his government to respect Indian tenures in the South "as long as grass grows and water flows," by professing that he had no power to enforce these treaties against the nullifying acts of local mobs. Though he answered South Carolina's threat of secession on a tariff matter with a warning that he would send in troops, he was silent when its sister states defied an order of the Supreme Court, broke the nation's solemn promises, threatened to secede, and made no move to restrain the depredations of individuals upon Indian lands.

In effect he said, "See, my Red Brothers, you will be happier if you go away, though you need go only of your own accord." His exact and strangely self-laudatory language is in a state document which speaks of "an ample district west of the Mississippi" where the red men, upon removal, could "raise up an interesting commonwealth to perpetuate the race and to attest the humanity and justice of this government."

The project, in a word, was that the nation was not itself to break faith; this was to be done by the states, and by what might be called the third degree. It is true that large blocks of Indian lands lay between white settlements, and that only over treaty-stipulated roads could these settlements have direct communication with each other. A real problem might have been solved by recognizing Indian culture and providing for a gradual absorption of these civilized communities into the body politic. Or it might have been solved by an honest abrogation of the federal treaties which gave the red men indefeasible title to the soil. The worst possible method was that which was followed. With Jackson looking on, rapacious men who coveted not only the Indian lands but all that was upon them—houses, crops, horses, and cattle—were able to get most of what they wanted. This was effected through state laws which reduced free red men almost to the level of black slaves, through the corrupt process of local courts, and through mob activities which anticipated the Ku Klux Klan.

When once the tribes were started westward, other palefaces—whisky-vending traders, contractors who furnished frozen potatoes, adventurers with eyes on the small commutation allowances given the fugitives—continued the work of spoliation. Yet the loss of their goods and chattels meant less to the tribesmen than that they were leaving the land in which their people had lived for centuries; for they were a settled folk with far less of the nomad in them than in the generation of white men which decried them as wandering hunters.

They lost their ancestral homes in the South, and the government of their white masters gained nearly a hundred thousand square miles in Georgia, Alabama, and Mississippi, paying two or three cents an acre for land which it resold to settlers for two or three dollars an acre. It looked like quite a bargain, but was it? With the forced removal a new strain entered the American nature, to warp it and work evil in the generations to come. This was the ingrained habit of trying to get something for nothing, whether by fraud or violence or both.

Most but not all of the Southern Indians made part of the journey on the Arkansas. Much depended on the stage of the river, the seaworthiness of the boats which bore them, and the mood of the deported peoples themselves when traders got to them and plied them with firewater—against which they had no usage to build up resistance. The story tells of halts at sand bars with the red men disembarking to lighten the boats and embarking again in deeper water; of protracted camps in the woods when cholera or smallpox had stricken the migrants, or government rations had failed to come; of cross-country treks in oxcarts when the river was down; of runaway flights of parties who subsisted on bear, deer, and other game in the swamps of Arkansas while they trended westward. The easternmost tribes had a journey of seven hundred miles before them. Most of the exiles were from three to five months on the way.

Forced migration began with the Choctaws in 1830, and ended with the Seminoles in 1843. The other tribes were the Creeks, Chickasaws, and Cherokees. Bad management on the part of the nation's civilian agents aggravated the woes of the departing peoples. Expeditions were undertaken too late or too early, so that winter found the half-clad fugitives—one government blanket to a family!—on the road. Men, women, and children used to open-air living were packed so closely on boats as to invite pestilence. Of the Cherokee nation alone, four thousand died during the exodus.

A motley fleet of boats was engaged in the removal. Most ambitious were the keelboats which bore a party of Cherokees down the Tennessee River. They were one hundred and thirty feet long with two-story structures upon them, stoves inside, and five hearths for cooking upon their roofs. A number of flatboats were used, some of them eighty feet long. These, of course, could go only downstream. Going up the Arkansas, they were in tow of steamboats, as were many of the keelboats. The names of steamboats, as set down here and there in Foreman's authoritative narrative of the removal, add up to nearly forty: *Archimedes, Black Hawk, Cavalier, Cleopatra, Elk, Erin, Farmer, Far West, George Guess, Harry Hill, Itaska, John Nelson, Lamplighter, Lewis Cass, Little Rock, Liverpool, Majestic, Meridian, Monmouth, Newark, North St. Louis, Ottawa, President, Reindeer, Renown, Rodney, Smelter, Swan, Tecumseh, Thomas Yeatman, Vesper, Victoria, Volant, Walter Scott, William Gaston.* Average tonnage of these boats was about one hundred and fifty.

Sometimes, when the steamboats moved out of the Mississippi, they entered the White River and later crossed over by the cut-off to the Arkansas. Because of snags and sand bars in an uncharted and unlighted channel, they traveled only by day, and seldom made much more than forty miles. Most of them ascended the Arkansas as far as Little Rock in the middle of the state. There many were replaced by steamboats of lighter draught which went up to Fort Smith, almost on the boundary of Oklahoma and three hundred and seventy miles from the river's mouth. Some were able to continue to Fort Gibson near the present city of Muskogee. Migration ended there and all around the Indians were the lands which had been set aside for them. The names of counties in the eastern half of Oklahoma—Sequoyah, Choctaw, Cherokee, Creek, Seminole, Osage, and Delaware—reveal where they and other exiled tribes from farther north found permanent habitation.

For once a woeful tale has a good ending. The Five Civilized Tribes settled down in eastern Oklahoma, re-established their ancient cultures, moved forward. Their unoccupied lands farther west they ceded to the nation, so that other and friendly tribes should have a home. Among these were the Cheyennes, Arapahoes, Kiowas, Comanches, Sacs and Foxes, Pawnees, Iowas, Kickapoos, Shawnees, Pottawatomies, Wichitas, Sioux, and Otoes. Oklahoma, a Choctaw word, means "land of the red man," and in a measure, so it is. It sent a red man to the Senate at Washington. Another red man from a neighboring state became Vice President. In the slow justice of time the Arkansas River had emerged as the highway to an enduring Indian civilization.

The second chapter the Arkansas wrote in the story of the Southwest was written before the railroads took over. This may well be called the Commerce of the Prairies, which is the name of a book written by Josiah Gregg, its best remembered figure. This was the movement of American men and goods (mostly drygoods) over the high plains to the desert emporium of Santa Fe. Alone of all the early routes westward, the Santa Fe Trail had a splash of exotic color, fetching up at a gay little outpost of civilization, instead of among the pines in gold-hoarding high sierras or by the waves of a blue, empty ocean.

The trail began at Independence on the Missouri River not far from the Kansas line. Many of the merchants, however, shipped their goods on the Arkansas to Fort Smith and there picked them up in their covered wagons. The rest, if they were well advised, bent their course sharply southward from Independence, and entering Indian Territory followed the valley of the Canadian River, main affluent of the Arkansas, clear to Santa Fe. There was a trickle of pack-horse trade as early as 1812 when golden reports, brought back by the Pike expedition, excited the imagination and cupidity of Americans. Not until 1824 were wagons used so that goods could go forward in quantity. From that time until a great railroad reached New Mexico's capital in 1880, the Santa Fe Trail was the scene of the most bizarre traffic in American history. Four countries had something to do with it: France, whose blockade of the Mexican coasts barred imports by sea and thus opened the way for the covered wagons to bring in their commodities; Spain, and then Mexico, whose petty governors and tax-collectors were at the far end of the trail; and the United States, under which its closing chapter was written.

Most of the goods carried over the trail were sent on down the valley of the Rio Grande to Chihuahua. The American merchants brought back from Santa Fe gold dust, peltries, coarse blankets and other Mexican weaves, and some Indian silverwork.

Best account of this trade is Gregg's *Commerce of the Prairies*. Beginning in May, 1831, he made eight different trips in as many years, the first as member of a caravan starting from Independence. It mustered two hundred men and a hundred wagons hauled by mules and oxen, dragged along two cannon, and had "a wild and motley aspect." Merchandise was valued at two hundred thousand dollars. The route lay through unbroken prairie for five hundred miles, with no timber save stream-bordering cottonwoods.

Few tents were taken along. The men slept in buffalo

robes under the serene skies of the plains, and liked it.
They chased bison herds, feasted on their humps, and
cured the beef in the dry, pure desert air. They held par-
leys with large bands of plausible, horse-stealing, wife-
loaning Comanches. They rode through streets of vast
prairie-dog towns. They were pelted by storms of hail-
stones larger than hen's eggs. With emotion they saw the
snowy summits of the Rockies appear on the horizon.

At the end was Santa Fe, a mile in air, with its wide
market place, its sunburned palace, its intimate patios
shadowed with almond trees and festooned with strings of
red peppers. There was a fandango in which reboso-draped,
jewel-bedecked, slim-ankled señoritas danced with the
traveled merchants. Thus a prairie epic came to its merry
close.

Less than a generation after the wagons of traders began
to move along the Santa Fe Trail, the third chapter de-
scribing the Arkansas' services was written when the wagons
of gold seekers appeared there and on routes roughly
parallel. A great migration set in. Though the fact is but
scantily noted, half or more than half of it started by water
—in steamboats and flatboats down the Ohio, up or down
the Mississippi to the Arkansas, and up that river to the
edge of the Indian country, where the land journey began.
There were times when overloaded packets discharged passengers almost daily at the frontier towns of Fort Smith or
near-by Van Buren after a trip of from four to seven days
up the Arkansas. In a single season fifteen thousand men,
most of whom had been carried up that waterway, were
toiling along the haggard Gila River route, which crossed
the desert from Santa Fe westward.

While more gold seekers followed the northern track—
the Oregon Trail—up the valley of the unnavigable Platte,

the southern route, up the Arkansas and along the valley of the tributary Canadian to Santa Fe, had things in its favor. Spring came earlier on the high plains, and that meant pasture for the livestock; with April the wagons started rolling. Another advantage was that the track between the two forts of the Canadian was a natural highway that on a fairly uniform grade climbed slowly toward the Rockies.

The wagon folk went westward in companies under officers many of whom had seen service in the Mexican War. Some companies had fieldpieces, all had traveling forges to shoe their beasts and shrink and reset wagon tires; at times they stopped to make charcoal for these prairie smithies. Cows were taken along for milk and butter. Horses and mules were bought when needed from the plumed banditti of the plains.

Adventure moved westward with the wagons. When a creek was to be crossed, its vertical banks were dug down and the stream was forded with due avoidance of quicksands; or boats were improvised of caulked wagon beds, or rafts made by buoying up wagon beds with empty barrels. Buffalo herds were drawn upon for fresh meat; deer, turkeys, prairie chickens, and jack rabbits varied the travel fare; wild June grapes were a welcome table item. Mesquite beans provided feed for cattle. Sometimes hay was cut, cured, and twisted for use in the desert stretches beyond. Letters to people back home were put in forked sticks for returning travelers to deliver. Messages and route information were scribbled on the bleached bones and skulls of oxen. At night in the pilgrim corrals, fiddles played and people sang and danced.

Though slower than horses and mules, oxen bore up better; and besides, Indians were under no temptation to steal them since buffaloes, their wild cousins, were to be had anywhere and their flesh was sweeter. As this strange trek proceeded and ways grew worse, men cast aside their burdens—turning wagons into carts by dropping one pair of wheels, shifting from carts to pack horses, discarding tents, stoves, utensils, harness, guns, books, even bacon. At Santa Fe they found desert markets, fiestas, beguiling señoritas, and their hearts lightened. What lay ahead, which was grim, has no place here, for it was along streams that flowed to the Pacific, when they flowed at all.

CHAPTER VIII

STEAMBOAT DAYS

FOR some while on our back track from New Orleans we seemed to be riding into summer instead of away from it. Balmy airs played about us, a blue sky bent overhead, flaming sunsets succeeded each other, and the night brought out stars never seen except on water and in lonely places. The crescent moon drifted among them. One evening it was pale green. When I walked the decks I had to pick my way around the legs of passengers sprawled out in quasi-summer attire. One man, I noted, wore congress gaiters.

The warm spell stayed with us because we were going upstream, against a strong current and high water, and we therefore went slow—eight or nine miles an hour instead of fifteen. Somewhat we eluded the current by hugging the banks and availing ourselves of slack water behind the bends. This meant zigzagging, for they were first on one side and then on the other. An earlier traveler counted nearly four hundred bends between New Orleans and St. Louis; but the river has straightened out some of these, and army engineers others. Now it is hundreds of miles shorter, and not a mile of it—says Mark Twain—in the same place as when De Soto discovered it in 1541. A shifty vagabond of many beds, as well as a ruthless old man, is the Father of Waters.

We were close enough to shore to see muskrat traps there, and surmise that the eyes of Cajun trappers surveyed us from the thickets. Water from the winding bayous was in the woods nearly everywhere, and out of it came a continual frog chorus.

Somewhere in Louisiana an impenetrable fog laid its spell on the river, and we moved over to the bank, thrust our bow into it, and remained there for four hours of the morning. There was plenty of fallen timber in the woods, and logs and poles are useful in many ways on a steamboat. So the crew set up a stepladder against the bank, and going ashore began to garner things in the forest. After breakfast many of us followed them. We were in a plantation of sycamores, the "broad-leafed planes" of the classic poets; some of the leaves, scattered over hummocks and hollows, were nearly a foot each way. I followed a bird note strange to me, but never set eyes on the singer. Others brought in sprays of blooming blackberry.

When another dense fog came on at night we took refuge among the willows and owls on the Arkansas bank, let down the gangplank, and unblinded the boat, which thereafter was a blaze of light in a wilderness without habitation. A few passengers went ashore again, stumbled over roots and logs, and soon returned. Pertinent was the comment of one of the colored maids, for the gangplank was a two-way road, up which the night could send its creatures.

"I'se afraid," she said. "S'pose a b'ar came aboard!"

It looked to me like bear country.

Such incidents served to heighten a sense of fellowship, since whatever happened to the boat happened to all of us. The packet had become a floating village with its own resources of entertainment. As I look back, I am amused and a little touched by that chapter of intimate friendliness. Save for logrolling and corn husking, we did about everything that people used to do in the back settlements: dancing the Paul Jones, with Captain Tom calling the turns, engaging in a poetry contest, holding a spelling bee, giving concerts, putting on a spirited minstrel show, improvising a church-singing service. On other occasions there were harmonica solos, piano duets, tap dances, parlor magic, palm readings, a grab-bag evening, a mock wedding in which the bride carried a bouquet of jimson weeds, a ladies' dress-up night, a masquerade ball. The black cabin boys and maids obliged with a good concert. Four of their numbers that I thought quite in keeping were "Lighthouse, Shine on Me," "River, Stay Away From My Door," "Give Me That Old-Time Religion," and "Lights Out."

Of course there were coteries. Members of the Kiwanis and Rotary clubs had one luncheon to themselves. There was a group of young matrons meeting daily in a small cabin in the stern of the texas who insisted on calling themselves The Rear End Club. My own routine was to walk five miles daily on deck alone, with supplemental mileage to music and of course with a partner at night. After dark, however, when canvas blinds shut off the outside world so that the pilot could steer without being dazzled by the steamboat's lights, the social atmosphere broadened to include all.

My preference among my companions may have been the Kentucky farmer whose mule, as already noted, listened with him when a steamboat whistled. As he confided to me, he had been "killt" by another mule, which pouched its hoof squarely in his face, had been "drownded" three times, had fallen off a bridge, and once had gone down with a snagged steamboat. These things happened when he was rousting on the river from St. Louis to New Orleans and along the lagoons of Louisiana—all before he was twenty-three years of age. Sometimes he got a job ashore, but whenever a steamboat whistle blew he was off again. For the last fifty years he had been a farmer above Louisville, but once more the river had got him. He was having the time of his life, and so was his charming, white-haired wife. "Such good people aboard," he said, "I'm learning a lot from them." I told him he was learning us a lot more than we could teach him.

However, I interrupted his tale of going down with a sinking steamboat. "On Bayou Teche," he began, "we ran into a floating cypress log five feet in diameter."

"Hold on!" I said. "That log was in the water. How did you know it was five feet thick?"

"Wait, and you'll find out," said the veteran farmer, and proceeded with his narrative.

The log which struck them had a projecting snag and the boat set it rolling across its own course. Every time the snag came up it punched a hole in the little stern-wheeler. There were four holes in the hull, each fifteen feet from its neighbor. Divide fifteen feet, the indicated circumference of the log by three, and you get its diameter, which was five feet.

"Your point is well taken," I conceded, and the farmer kept on.

The captain drove his sinking craft into a slough on the prairie side of the bayou, where it rested on the bottom, only the pilothouse showing above water. A wrecking crew, summoned from New Orleans, hauled it out on the sloping shore. "Every time a hole came up," said the Kentuckian, "water poured out—fishes, too. Some of them were that long," and his hands sketched finny creatures perhaps half as long as the log was broad.

Our boat newspaper kept a daily record of the craft which we met, the people who had come aboard or gone off at way ports, and the birthdays of passengers. Among its bits of quoted miscellany was the following Morality, credited to Mark Twain: "Do right; you will thereby please some and astonish the rest." It was announced that half-gallon cans of sorghum could be had at the boat's store; that in the office was a scrapbook filled with menus from famous New Orleans restaurants to refresh our memories, and that Natchez had a syllabub worthy of special note—something compiled from milk and cream, to which rum or sherry was added for flavor, and a red-hot poker was plunged in for fiery drama. At the end of the cruise the paper reported that we had eaten, among other things, a ton and a half of potatoes, two tons of beef, sixteen lambs, five calves, five hundred chickens ("a whole barnyard") and four hundred pounds of bacon.

When we rounded Plum Point, still as in Twain's day a thing difficult to do, our newspaper recorded that towboats have to take soundings to measure the depths there. The leadsman heaves forward a weighted line, on which is a series of markers, and counts the markers as the line slips through his fingers. His chant has a different tone for each depth, so that the pilot understands even if passengers do not. He may be saying Mark Twain, which is twelve feet; or Half Twain, which is fifteen feet; or Deep Four, twenty-four feet; or No Bottom, which is more than that.

Anybody who travels the Lower Mississippi is sure to hear from somebody the sagas of four noted river boats— the *Natchez,* the *Robert E. Lee,* the *Minotaur,* and the *Grand Republic.* For the twelve-hundred-mile race of the two first-named packets from New Orleans to St. Louis, in 1870, I might take as text almost any one of twenty-nine stanzas of a ballad written a while ago by Captain Joe Brown. For example:

> On board the Lee they plain could see
> The Natchez' roaring fire,
> And as they pitched the rosin in
> Could see the steam get higher.

This was the country's biggest sporting event and even in London and Paris large sums of money were wagered. Both boats were built on the Ohio and commanded by Ohio River masters, each of them a Kentuckian with hot sporting blood. The *Natchez* was Cincinnati-made. The *Lee* was begun downstream on the Indiana side, but when the Hoosiers learned what name it was to bear, it had to be towed across the river to escape their wrath. In the great race it reached St. Louis six hours and a half ahead of its rival. River men say, however, that the other was the faster boat and lost out because it made its usual stops to handle freight and passengers, while the rival declined all way traffic and in addition to pine knots—which both boats burned—had a supply of spoiled fat bacon, rosin, and tallow candles to make hotter steam. Yet the *Lee's* time of three days, eighteen hours and fourteen minutes from port to port has never been equaled. For reasons of sentiment nearly everybody along the Mississippi wanted the race to end as it did anyway.

The steamboat *Minotaur* had a legendary history in keeping with its ancient and forbidding name. Because of the legend, Mississippi navigators used to say that any boat the name of which begins with the letter M—thirteenth in the alphabet—was under an evil spell. According to the story told by Julius Chambers, two well-dressed strangers, calling themselves Louisiana planters, boarded the boat at Memphis on the down trip, and engaged Captain Durkin in draw poker. When four kings were dealt him, he bet all his money and his quarter-interest in the boat, only to be confronted with four aces. Signing a bill of sale for his share of the boat, he retired to his stateroom and shot himself. The note he left declared: "A man who would bet his last dollar on four kings doesn't deserve standing room on earth."

After the *Grand Republic* was launched following the Civil War, a flamboyant age had no direction to go except backward, for this was the last word. Down the long cabin with its fluted columns, fretted arches, and overhead lights, the passenger looked as down the nave and aisles of some great cathedral. An insignificant item will save further description: the crew included a lamp cleaner whose sole task was to take care of the chandeliers. This was the biggest, finest, and probably fastest of all packets, but its engines were so powerful that the captain never dared to open up and find out. For good reasons it was known as the Calendar Boat. It was three hundred and sixty-five feet long, and that is the number of days in the year; fifty-two feet wide, the number of weeks in the year; twelve feet deep in the hull, the number of months in the year. In honor of the seven days in the week there were seven decks. The floor of the main cabin was covered by a Brussels carpet three hundred feet long and thirty feet wide, specially woven in Belgium in one piece for the boat. It cost forty dollars a square yard.

From the decks of the *Gordon C. Greene* we saw less showy craft come and go, mainly by day. Ships that pass in the night and speak one another in passing may be "only a signal shown and a distant voice in the darkness," if they pass at sea. On the river, as we found, there was a little more—a vague blur of light, the jangle of bells, comradely whistle blasts; but we never learned the names or trades of those boats. Of all we met in the daytime, going or coming, I remember the towboats *Slack Barrett, Tennessee, Louisiana, J. D. Ayres,* and *Jacona;* the ferryboat *George Prince* and the steamboat *Tennessee Belle,* both at Natchez; the harbor excursion boat *Capitol* at New Orleans; the ferryboat *Lorrene,* which came alongside at the Arkansas town of Helena to take off two passengers; the army towboat

Coiner, and the side-wheeler *Willow,* another government boat, which tends shore lights on the lower river. There were also several treasury boats, survivals of the prohibition era, when a fleet of small, fast vessels patrolled long reaches of timbered shore behind which the smoke of illicit stills was rising.

With the *Coiner* we came as near to a race as army traditions would sanction. At Vicksburg it beat us out of the Yazoo River and got the start, hugging slack water along the shore and compelling us to battle the swift current in midstream. Again and again we drew abreast, and at last ahead; but then the meanderings of the channel gave it titular right to blow the passing whistle, and we fell back. "Just prior to press time," said our newspaper, "the *Coiner* disappeared through a newly dug chute and was seen no more."

Now and then we came upon flotillas of barges pushed by stout towboats and operated by two lines which carry most of the commerce of the river. The Mississippi Valley Barge Line, which bears cargo to and from New Orleans out of both Cincinnati and St. Louis, is owned by private capital. It has four towboats and a growing fleet of barges. The Federal Barge Line, which is government-owned, has twenty-seven towboats and numerous barges. Established in the World War to relieve freight congestion on the railroads, its first service was between St. Louis and New Orleans. Now its trades are up the Mississippi to St. Paul, up the Illinois and connecting waterways to Chicago, up the Missouri to Kansas City, and out of the Mississippi and into the Gulf eastward as far as Mobile.

Our first scheduled stop upstream was at the Louisiana town of Plaquemine. Here an ordinary packet can pass by lock out of the Mississippi and reach the Gulf by way of a canal, a lake, a bayou, and another river. A ferryboat laden with good cypress boards came out and we took them on. So other steamboats do, for these cost only one-third as much there as in Cincinnati, and because they do not rot in water they come handy in mending stern timbers. They were put aboard by lean, tanned youths with black, coarse hair. When I asked if they were Cajuns, they demurred; the Acadian country, they said, was "as much as eighteen mile away." But passengers were skeptical.

The fate of Kaskaskia, old Illinois territorial capital, sunk for a generation beneath the Mississippi's waters, was also that of the town of Napoleon, which stood on the point where the Arkansas comes in, and is now lying in the bottom of the river; in the same watery grave, as heretofore noted, is Natchez-under-the-Hill. When we passed Vidalia, a sweet and venerable little town on the Louisiana shore across from Natchez, we were bade to look at it twice, or thrice, for none of us might ever see it again. The cut-off above Natchez doomed it, and this had to be made, for the river was undermining the bluffs of that old Spanish town. Vidalia may end in the next flood.

Here and elsewhere we watched the army's unending battle with the river. At first individual planters, building detached levees to protect their own holdings, had to do this alone. But by 1879 people got the thought that as the Mississippi carried off the waters of the country, its control was the national concern. After that, government engineers used all the devices they could think of. They built wider and higher levees—and the 1927 flood burst them. They ordained the nine-foot channel above Baton Rouge, and endeavor to maintain it by snagging and dredging and taking weekly soundings to locate and remove hidden bars. To narrow and deepen the channel, they built fences and retards, silt collecting behind them and advancing the shores. They revetted the banks against caving by means of mattresses woven from willow branches and held down with rocks, or made of asphalt and concrete. They created spillways through which surplus water could pass and so lower the crest of a flood; these worked well in the 1937 flood. Also, they established cut-offs.

Those cut-offs are a matter of debate among army engineers. If, for example, you cut a new channel only two miles long across a bend twenty-two miles around, you shorten the river twenty miles; but if in that journey around the bend it dropped half a dozen feet, it has to make the same drop thenceforth in two miles. That means fast water in the cut, above the cut, and below it, with a rapidly emptying river; it means that the flood hazard is abated in the valley above but augmented in the valley below, and in dry seasons there is likely to be a channel possibly too shallow for big boats. It is like leading a road straight up a hill instead of around it.

Through the Caulk Point cut-off across Monterey Bend we had shot like an arrow on our way down; thereafter for a while we ran along at twenty-three miles an hour. With a sense of drama we entered it again on our way up, for we knew what it had done a fortnight before to the Federal Barge Line boat *Vicksburg*, which entered it pushing a tow. "Go round about," said the river, which, you remember, was the maxim of the Great Boyg, god of Ways That Are Crooked, in Ibsen's *Peer Gynt*. Shoving the flotilla back into the main channel, it forced it on a humiliating sixteen-mile ride around the bend to a point that was but little more than a mile away.

Government dredges had made a ditch a hundred feet or so wide across the neck the preceding November, and left the rest to the river, which takes years to widen, deepen, and round out a new stretch of waterway.

Every boat helps in this task, for its waves do things to

the crumbling banks. We watched them as our packet moved in. Loosened earth slid in small streams from under the turf. The naked roots of naked, nodding willows over-hung the swirling water. Then a tall tree, wearing the green leafage of spring, toppled over and fell in with a loud crash, the spray flying far above it, and just above the spray two startled wild ducks. Amid equal tumult a second tree smote the turbid water.

Passengers crowded to the bow to watch a drama's denoue-ment—the final struggle of the packet against the main current of the Mississippi where the latter swept into the cut-off from what seemed a higher level. Looking at the surface, I thought we were going fast. Looking at the shore, it was another story. "I could outwalk the boat," I de-clared. Over whirlpools that would have stood a rowboat on its end we crawled along—just the word, for there I could have crawled as fast on my hands and knees—and when at last we swept back into the river, a cheer went up. It had taken us twenty-five minutes to go a fraction more than a mile.

Though our packet went on to Cincinnati, the cruise lasting twenty days, this is the point where I think Mark Twain would have ended his account of it. Anyway, I do.

CHAPTER IX

RIVER PORT

FOUNTAIN SQUARE is the traditional center of Cincinnati life. Once it was covered by a great, fly-haunted market house. Only by replacing it with a fountain could the city get rid of the vested rights of forty butchers. It did a good job of it, filling the square with the murmur of falling water, satisfying the eye with a tasteful arrangement of figures done in a refined baroque style. The fountain was made in Munich. Most beautiful of its four groups of figures is that of a woman half unclad leading a naked boy to the bath. There is a scandalous tradition that the model for the woman was Lola Montez, the Irish adventuress who became mistress of King Louis of Bavaria and by her escapades caused an insurrection, practically dancing him off his throne. It is more to the point that the south panel of the pedestal—that facing toward the Ohio—shows a side-wheeler lying along a river shore. Thus through the generations the city declares its awareness of the forces that brought it into being.

One of these forces—robust and romantic—was that of the foremost naturalist of America, who quested along rivers on a number of which, more than a century later, I traveled myself. When Audubon paused for a while to resume family life and get in some needed cash by running a mill or a store, or painting portraits, or stuffing birds and animals, it was at river towns—Cincinnati, Louisville, Shippingport, and Henderson, all on the Ohio, and at New Orleans. For a while he was employed in a natural history museum in Cincinnati. There were no railroads then, no good roads; so he journeyed by canoe, flatboat, broadhorn, steamboat, on muleback, or afoot. Though he was often desperately hard up, perhaps he lived more joyously, and certainly saw more things worth seeing, than any other American of his time. The Ohio Valley has rightful claims on his fame.

I have not been able to take the river altogether for granted, as men are wont to take familiar objects. For years I have looked out upon it daily from the newspaper building where I worked; a glance would tell me whether it was rising or falling, and how much; from the sheen upon it I knew what sort of sky was overhead. Sometimes when I was downtown at night I descended to the levee to see the dark craft huddled there, the lights of the Kentucky shore, a moon riding the water. The bovine note of a fog-bound packet was a welcome sound in my sleep, and the wild music of a calliope, heard from near or far, always did things to me. In other parts of this narrative I have done as all river writers—and all steamboats—do, which is to start from where they are and go somewhere else. In the present chapter I shall stay where I am.

But the double rows of hooting steamboats that once thronged the levee front are heard from no more. Things seem quiet, a deceptive quiet. Nowadays freight comes and goes, not in packets but in barges pushed by towboats, and towboats do not advertise their presence with whistles. Last year's tonnage on the Ohio was five times as great as that in the World War year of 1918 and almost equal to tonnage through the Panama Canal. How this could be was demonstrated years before when the *Sprague* went down the river with sixty barges, containing seventy thousand tons of coal. It would have taken a hundred and twenty good-sized packets to carry that cargo. Nowadays, sixty-three boats of major size come and go in the harbor; two showboats, one passenger boat, one excursion boat, one Coast Guard cutter, all the rest freighters.

There are four common carrier barge lines, each with its towboats and a cluster of barges; four coal lines, the fleets of which come down from the West Virginia mines; two lines which carry oil and gasoline; three steel lines with their barges; seven towboats which propel cement barges; a coke boat, and a general freight line with four steamboats, two of them converted packets. Other towboats with cargoes of steel for the lower Mississippi pass through the harbor without stopping.

Gideon's Band, by George W. Cable, speaks of a wharfboat at Natchez in 1852. Civil War pictures show small wharfboats tied at Cincinnati's Public Landing. These amphibious craft came into being in the first generation of steamboats. They are both passenger stations and warerooms, in which you may find apples, potatoes, cabbages, tropical fruits, farm implements, baled hay, chicken feed, groceries, tobacco sticks, cars, now and then the household goods of a family moving by river, or even live hogs, cattle, and mules. Wharfboats are the answer to two uncertainties—that of the rivers and that of the packets. If rivers kept at the same level, stationary docks would suffice. If the old-time packets could have kept their schedules, and kept off sand bars and away from snags, passengers who had come in from the backwoods would not have had to wait for indefinite periods at the landings. But sometimes a river rose a dozen feet a day. The wharfboat, moored to shore, could rise with it, and put out a gangplank over which goods and people moved. Sometimes night brought no packet. So a few of the larger wharfboats had a second story with beds for passengers.

Though the packets are fading from the picture, perhaps the greatest of all wharfboats lies at Cincinnati's Pub-

lic Landing, and it is new. Long and low and wide—three
hundred and sixty feet, by seventy-five—it looks like a shed,
a barn, a ranch house, yet it draws less than four feet of
water. At one end in a sort of balcony (granary would be
a more descriptive term) are the offices of the Greene line.
This great floating dock stands for a fortunate circum-
stance repeated nowhere else on the inland rivers. The
cities of Cincinnati and Louisville, one hundred and twenty
miles downstream, are only a night's run from each other
by the freighters, and there is plenty of business at each
end so that boats come and go with full cargoes.

There is a sort of barge harbor in the West End of
Cincinnati. From the deck of a towboat I looked upstream
over a fleet of barges that were taking on or discharging
miscellaneous cargo from or to the ports of the Mississippi,
and to another fleet of barges laden with West Virginia
coal. Looking downstream, I saw two Africans cooking
something at a fire on the bank, and beyond them a cluster
of shanty boats, with shirts and overalls fluttering on the
clothesline.

I had been on a number of steamboats, but never on a
towboat, barring the wooden craft on which I had traveled
two Southern streams. That was why I made a visit to the
river and the Mississippi Valley Barge Line. The *Ohio*
had just completed a fourteen-day run from New Orleans.
Descending the mud bank by a sketchy flight of wooden
steps, I went aboard, stopping on the way to look through
a flotilla of barges, painted a torpedo-boat gray, which lay
between the boat and the bank. One was a blacksmith shop
with anvil and bellows, where men were shaping hot iron.
Another was a wood-working plant. A third had machine
tools. These were the repair shops of the line.

Being an all-steel boat, the *Ohio* is not as picturesque as
the old wooden packets, on which I have ridden. It could

not be. They were gaudy and gilded, and rose high out of the water like a swan; the towboat is more on the flat-backed duck pattern. Yet it is a handsome boat in its compact, efficient way.

It does not carry passengers, nor freight. It just pushes barges in front of it, and therefore its living room space, for officers and crew—twenty-eight in all—is limited. But I noted a small lounge, well-appointed sleeping rooms with baths, a radio office, a laundry, messrooms for officers and crew, the cook's galley, ice rooms where meat and vegetables and dairy products are kept, filters to provide drinking water, and a glassed-in pilothouse which was true to river tradition in that it had a high chair, and an elevated leather-cushioned observation bench of the sort that always makes me think of a bootblack's stand.

This is what is called the tunnel type of towboat, steam driven, but burning oil instead of coal. Its twin propellers operate in tunnels in the stern, on the principle of an outboard motor, and there are four rudders. Two hundred feet long, forty feet in beam, and with engines of two thousand horsepower, it makes the down trip to New Orleans with a fleet of barges in seven days, and takes twice that long to come back. Its usual rate of speed is somewhat less than that of the passenger packets. Stops are made at way points to pick up loaded barges of tobacco. No freight is discharged until Memphis is reached. There are three other towboats, all bearing the names of states; every three hours they get in radio touch with the home office.

Looking along the shore, I saw the work of unloading proceed. At a tipple in the distance, clamshell buckets were lifting the coal from thousand-ton barges and carrying it to hoppers, whence it was taken away in railroad cars or trucks. Midstream, a barge piled high with sulphur, perhaps from Texas, was going up the river. Nearer at

hand a monster crane, which had been used at Muscle
Shoals, reached out one arm a hundred feet or more,
picked up carriers full of boxed merchandise, took them
to the side of railroad cars in the river-rail terminal, and
returned the carriers empty to the barge below. From the
terminal's upper level, elevators lowered electric trucks to
the very doors of barges. This process of loading and unloading does not dispense with the roustabout, but it does
dispense with his gangplank trips to and from the shore.
He still rousts, but not about.

I explored one of the steel barges. With a covered deck
over the hold, and seeming rather like a double-decked
box-car, it will carry close to three hundred tons. Any
number of barges can be grouped in a streamline pattern.
A barge fleet is lashed tightly to towing knees in the bow
of the boat, so that everything moves as one piece, like
log rafts in the yesterdays. There is nothing wrong with
all this, except the name towboat, which pushes instead of
pulls. What might happen if one of the tugboats you see
in New York harbor should start down the Ohio, pulling
a bunch of barges at the end of a long rope, would be just
too bad.

There remains one boat to be described, one which perhaps I have left till last because of the lowly status it
occupies in the sight of the towboats, barges, and wharfboats that ply a serious trade on the waters of the Ohio.

Now, a shanty, you will agree, is a house of sorts, but a
house need not be a shanty. So with floating dwellings. A
shanty boat is a houseboat, but a houseboat may not be a
shanty boat, and usually is not. The matter depends somewhat on the social rank of the tenant, somewhat on whether
he has a steady job, and more on the interior furnishings
of his mind than on those of his craft. The distinction,

though often a bit vague, is important from the stand-
point of the law, for houseboats may dock anywhere along
both shores of Cincinnati harbor, while its bordering
cities deny their water fronts to shanty boats. In intervals
of law enforcement they are moored in outlying coves.

Their owners are nomad folk, and may be of pioneer
stock. Some are former hillmen from Kentucky. Others
are descended from men who pulled the sweeps on rafts
and flatboats, or earned day's wages at steamboat landings, or drifted down the rivers to find jobs in the sawmills that were cutting down and cutting up the virgin
forest. The shanty boatman is a casual workman who pays
no taxes and no rents, supplies his table with catfish taken
from the river, burns driftwood in his kitchen stove, and
equips his humble home, it may be, with chairs, bedstead,
a table, a clock, and perhaps a violin or guitar, which high
water has brought him. Sometimes he shoots a wild duck
or a tame hen. It is tradition that he raids the corn rows
and garden patches nearest the waters, and he has Biblical
sanction for doing so. Embodying the timeless paradox of
nomadic restlessness and a deep love of leisure, perhaps he
is a symbol of the river itself.

For what is left of Cincinnati's shipyard industry, one
must go down the Mississippi to Algiers, across the river
from New Orleans, and to the wharves of a steamship line
there which fell heir to it. No signs of it are left along the
stretch of Ohio's shore which runs east from the Public
Landing. Yet there in the preceding century boat yards
and sawmills covered miles of the water front, and back
of them were hotels which served the trade. At least four
seagoing vessels were built before 1850—a ship, a full-rigged
brig, and two barks. The arrival in England in 1845 of
the *Muskingum,* constructed farther upstream but clearing

from Cincinnati, seventeen hundred miles from the Gulf, caused British exclamations of amazement.

Steamboat building, while it lasted, was a high chapter in Cincinnati history. Launching its first packet in 1816, the city soon took a leading rank. In 1826, out of one hundred and forty-three steamboats on all the inland rivers, forty-eight were Cincinnati-made. In 1840 the local yards turned out thirty-three boats, in 1842 they turned out forty-five. The total runs into the hundreds. A few Cincinnati boats, built for the South American trade, went out of the Mississippi and essayed to cross the Gulf and the Caribbean; not all of them got across. A number were shipped in pieces and set up in foreign countries; more were designed in local lofts by skilled workmen who carried the plans abroad, constructing boats which plied the Amazon, the Orinoco, the Magdalena, the Volga, the Nile, and the Congo. The last Cincinnati-made steamboat of any consequence was the first *Island Queen,* built in 1896.

Cincinnati is the capital, in all matters pertaining to navigation and flood control, of what, to use an old term, might be called the Ohio Country. It covers fourteen states or parts of states, six of them on the Atlantic seaboard. The entire watershed of the Ohio—about two hundred and four thousand square miles—is in charge of army engineers stationed in the Queen City. This includes the big river, its eleven navigable affluents, and every small river, creek, or brook tributary thereto. The principal streams are the Allegheny, Monongahela, Muskingum, Kanawha, Little Kanawha, Big Sandy, Kentucky, Green, Barren, Cumberland, and Tennessee.

The city also is one of the five district offices of the watershed. Three hundred engineers are stationed there. Its limits have pictorial names—from "a point below Big

Sandy River to Lonesome Hollow Creek," which is nearly
two hundred and forty miles. The office built and operates
the eleven locks and dams in this stretch of the river. Removal of snags, dredging of bars, and maintaining a year-
round nine-foot channel are among its duties. So are flood-
control projects at the headwaters of streams, and clearing
obstructions at the mouths of certain small tributaries such
as Licking, in which high water from the parent river
sometimes creates a harbor navigable for three miles back.
At the edge of the city are marine ways and shipyards
where government boats are built, repaired, or stored, by
a force of something less than two hundred men. Cincinnati harbor is the twenty-seven miles of river between the
mouths of the two Miamis.

When the *Tom Greene* and *Betsy Ann* had their famous
race up the Ohio a few years ago, there were men aboard
to watch the boilers. They came from the Division of
Marine Inspection and Navigation which also has its head-
quarters in Cincinnati and covers the wide Ohio Country.
The local office is ninety years old. Besides keeping an eye
on such contests—which lately have been rare—it tests
boilers and lifeboats, inspects tank barges containing com-
bustible liquids, conducts fire drills on passenger boats,
holds trials after river accidents, and examines and licenses
pilots.

Four steamboats, one named *Grace Darling*, descended
the Ohio and Mississippi in 1846, laden with bacon, lard,
and lard oil for the New Orleans markets. I have seen the
insurance policy, written by a vanished Lexington, Kentucky, house for their cargoes. Romance invests this passage: "Touching the adventures and perils which the afore-
said insurance company is contented to bear, they are of
the rivers, seas, men-of-war, fires, enemies, pirates, rovers,

thieves, jettisons, letters of mart and counter-mart, sur-
prisals, takings at sea, arrests, restraints, and detainments
of all kings, princes or people, and all other perils, losses
and misfortunes, which have, or shall, come to the hurt,
detriment or damage of the said Goods and Merchandise."

This category of the hazards of inland navigation may
seem fantastic; yet there were thieves on the rivers, some
of the packets adventured the open seas, and not far ahead
was a great war in which many of them went down in battle. Modern policies use much the same terms, and boats
and cargoes are insured in every considerable river port.
The biggest house in this line is in Cincinnati. Boats which
it underwrites—they number thousands—operate on the
entire navigable length of the Ohio and Mississippi, the
Missouri from Sioux City to its mouth, the Arkansas from
Pine Bluff to its mouth, the Red from Alexandria to its
mouth. The founder of the line was born in a covered
wagon in what used to be called York State and had been
a steamboat captain.

Marine insurance, like steamboating itself, was once a
risky thing. There were no government lights, and there
were snags and sand bars and racing captains. An average
steamboat lasted scarcely four years. The Ohio, however,
was always the safest of rivers, boats in 1870 paying 8 per
cent insurance a year on their hulls, as against 11 on the
Mississippi, 15 on the Arkansas, 16 on the Missouri, and
17 on Red River. Now steel towboats on the Ohio pay
from 2 to 4 per cent.

The oldest packet policy I have seen, which assured
Daniel Greene, ancestor of the present Greene river family, for ten thousand dollars against loss of his *Isabella*,
appraised at fifteen thousand dollars, was written in 1828.
Another old policy recites the cargo items which the companies insured against loss. Some of these I copied: "salt,

saltpetre, alum, copperas, corn, all kinds of grain, seeds, peas, beans, cider, beer, ale, tobacco, pork, bacon, cheese, dry fish, vegetables and roots, pleasure carriages, household furniture, skins and hides, musical instruments, looking glasses, books and stationery, hemp, yarns, bagging, bale-rope, twine, flax, bread, teas and sugar, (brown, white and loaf.)" All these commodities are still insurable, still carried on the inland rivers.

CHAPTER X

ALONG THE WATER FRONT

THERE was only thirteen feet of water in the channel. So I knew why pilots speak of the Hill. Cincinnati was so far above that it seemed to be in another world, a world of dark building fronts, and luminous, unreal towers beyond them. A winding sawdust path, on which young women were moving, led down the hill to the river. On a darkling current the lights of two bridges, the street lights of two cities, were reflected. I followed the path and entered the showboat. As I sat at a window there, the glamor of familiar yet always strange settings enveloped me, preparing me for whatever glamor the floating theater had to offer in *Bertha, the Sewing Machine Girl*.

While I awaited the curtain I bought peanuts, good peanuts, from an aisle man whom I recognized later as the madhouse guard of the play. So did a lot of Young Things who filled the center section of the boat. This was a sorority rush party from the university. They were out for a good time and disposed to deride all the traffic of the play. They made quite a racket. In the intermission when Billy Bryant expressed surprise to find them there—"you were so quiet that I never guessed it"—perhaps they glimpsed the Great Truth of his showboat showmanship, which is that the real kidding is done on the other side of the footlights.

Bertha's bosom heaved and fell, and she never cracked a smile; and yet, if I mistake not, the joyous young woman in the entr'acte vaudeville who wore overlong skirts and flopped through an amusing song-and-dance act was none other than she. When the villain told her that she was

125

"The Girl That Men Forget," and sang the song to that effect (it's an Olympic burlesque memory), her reaction to his bathos was splendid.

So the show proceeded, and the sorority lassies cheered and booed and made the walls of the boat bulge whenever a Sentiment was emitted, which was pretty often. At two places the script of the play may have been tampered with by some ribald river hand. In one passage a suitor speaks to his girl of moonlight rides on the canals of Venice. He mentions sycamores, whippoorwills and snags; I have seen these along the Ohio but never on the Grand Canal. The other spot was a reference to the occupation of the millionaire father of the young man whom Bertha has secretly married while servant in his home. When the sire would break up this match, the younger man proclaimed, "Then I will no longer be the son-of-a-biscuit-maker." The line, which sounded vaguely familiar, was received with sorority shouts.

Of course, Bertha's husband was disowned by his rich father, her baby abducted, herself confined in a madhouse, and there were attempted stabbings and poisonings. Things might not have gone well but for Cheatham (that was Billy Bryant), who intervened when needed. His appearance came to be expected, and once when seemingly delayed the sorority crowd shouted: "Cheatham, Cheatham! Bring on Cheatham!" It was quite an evening.

Descending Cincinnati's Broadway, I turned to the left at the Public Landing, walked across a number of beached floats which belonged to a canoe harbor, turned to the right, and followed a rude pathway of ashes down the mud flats. This fetched up at the river where I went aboard a waiting steamboat. It was the Coast Guard cutter *Greenbrier*, a lighthouse tender until July, 1939, when that

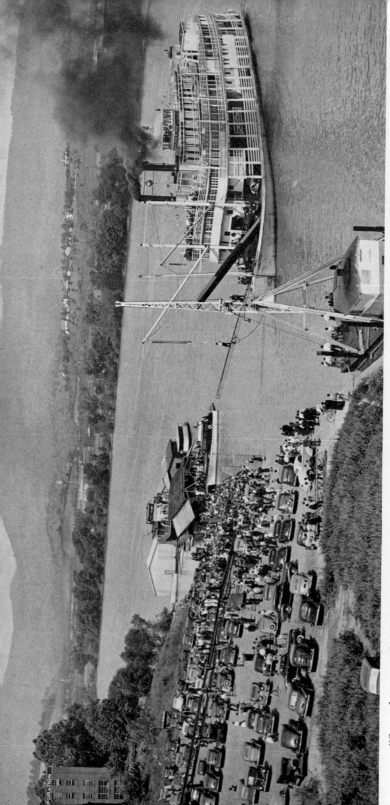

"Steamboat comin'!"—1941 version. Here the venerable packet *Golden Eagle* blows for a landing while the entire population of this Tennessee river town turns out to see the fun. Note the roustabout on the landing stage which will be lowered as soon as the steamer is made fast to the river bank.

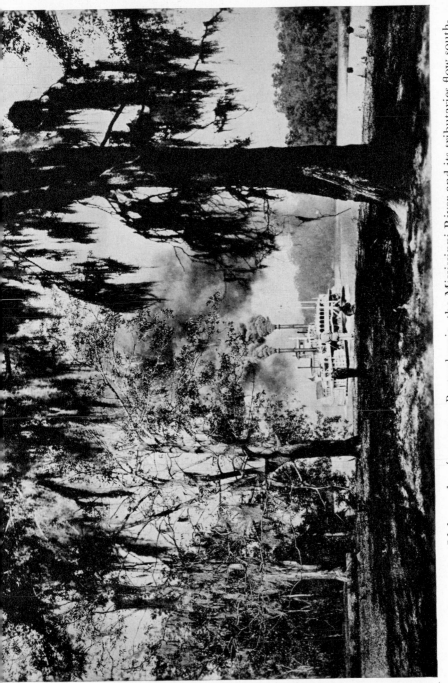

From as far west as Idaho and as far east as Pennsylvania, the Mississippi River and its tributaries flow southward down the valley to New Orleans and the sea.

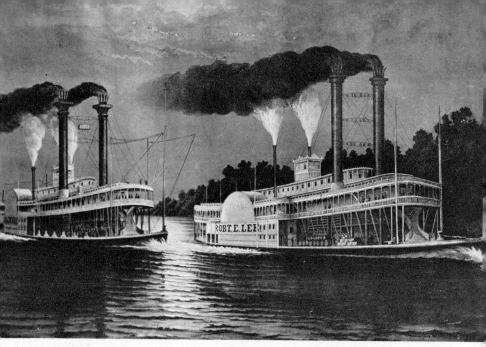

The famous race of the *Natchez* and the *Robert E. Lee*. It was one of the country's biggest sporting events, and has been recorded in both song and story. The race was from New Orleans to St. Louis, and was won by the *Lee,* whose time of three days, eighteen hours and fourteen minutes has never been equalled.

The *Gordon C. Greene* at Natchez, Mississippi. She carries a mixed cargo up and down both the Mississippi and the Ohio and makes summer and winter cruises which attract passengers who would relive the days of Mark Twain.

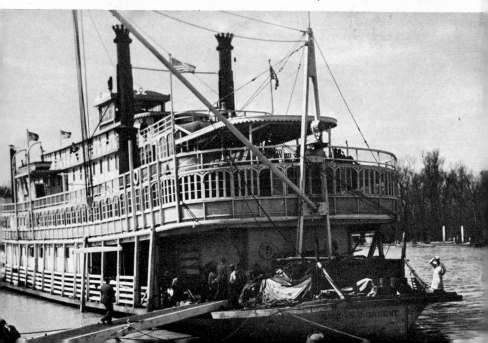

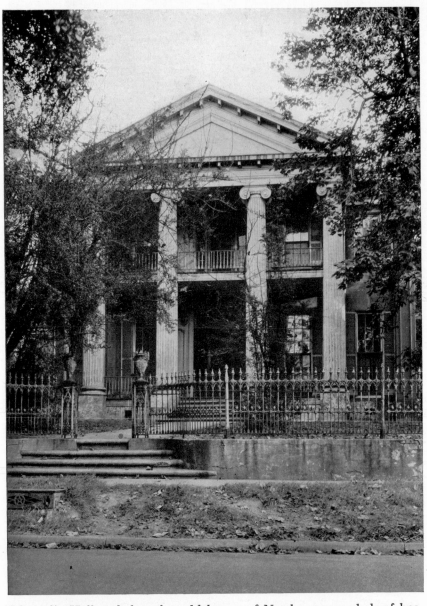

Magnolia Hall and the other old homes of Natchez are symbols of hospitality and with them are associated the names of many famous visitors.

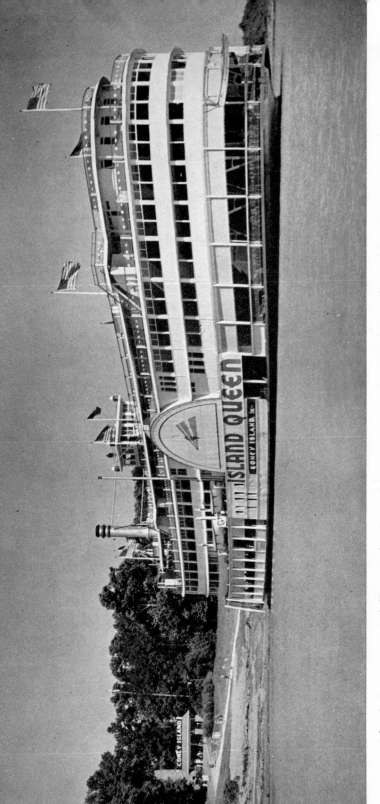

Island Queen—perennially popular excursion steamer on the Ohio. Complete with a jazz band, cafeteria and steam calliope, she is a source of joy and delight to Cincinnati's pleasure seekers.

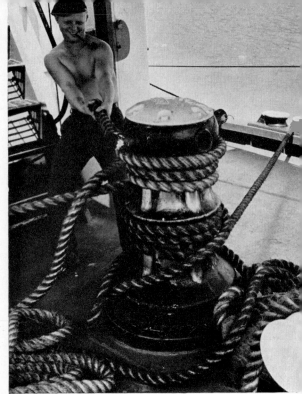

This tugboat deck man is winding the bow towlines around the capstan which towboats use to make fast their barges.

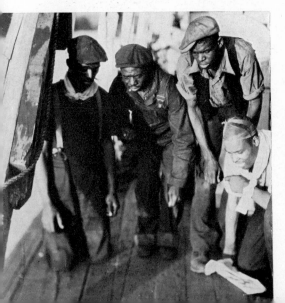

The river roustabouts contract to work twenty-four hours a day, seven days a week. Fortunately, however, there are idle moments. Here are some of them trying their luck at their favorite game.

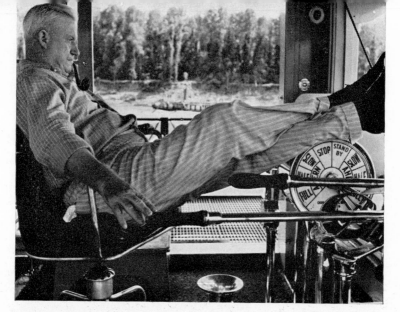

Forty years a pilot on the Mississippi and the Ohio, Captain Pete Brisco has seen life on the rivers change from the reckless, romantic days of the packets to the sober, steady freight traffic of today. Steering with levers, as is done in the modern motorships, is a simple matter to this old riverman who has handled the huge steering wheels of the old-time packets.

A sternwheeler has just passed through an Ohio River lock which this man is closing. There are forty-six locks on the Ohio, all but two of which are at movable dams so that there is "open river" down practically the whole stream for about six months of the year.

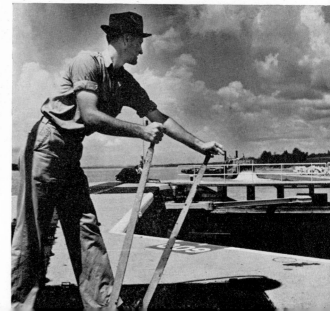

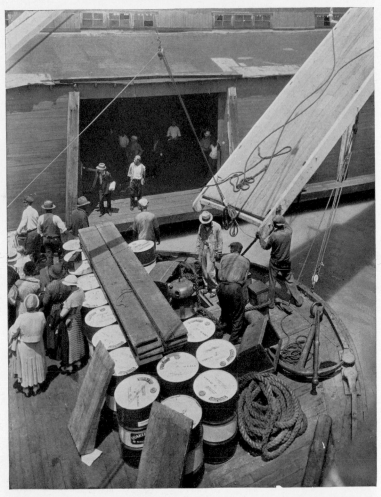

To the untrained eye, the loading of a river steamboat seems to be the worst kind of confusion. Actually, it is a highly organized procedure carried out with efficiency.

was swathed with sweet odors from down-river molasses
and up-river dried apples and peaches, sometimes with
the acrid smells of barnyard and poultry yard creatures.

Now and then the house would receive an entire steamboat load of dried fruits from the farms along the Big
Sandy and Little Kanawha. For a while it handled rags destined for the paper mills that lined the lower stretches of
the canal which ran from river to lake. Bales of feathers
came to it. Beeswax, a hundred tons a year, was an incident in its traffic. Ginseng, to bring up the virility of
the old men of China, was and is important. There were
years when the house handled five times the present American harvest of this strange root. Prices of ginseng have
varied within memory from twenty-eight dollars a pound
to thirty-seven cents; the 1940 figure was eight dollars a
pound.

The last time I was at the house, ginseng was not in
season and only piles of yellowseal—worth two dollars a
pound—stood for the pharmacopoeia of the pasture lots.
All else was raw furs, the odors of which were in every
room; men who work there grow to like the sharp smell
of skunkskins, which they say whets one's appetite and
tones up the system. The pelts handled were of small
creatures, brought in by trappers, farmers, and farm lads,
from the surrounding country—in the season just ended,
the skins of three thousand red foxes, five thousand gray
foxes, five thousand raccoons, and fifteen thousand muskrats. Perhaps there was a feral note in the trapper group,
an Indian among them, who sat around a stove in the
office.

Though for the most part rivers follow a narrow way,
the wide bottom lands on each side belong to them, and
periodically they assert title by occupancy. That is a flood.

Little rivers knock things around, big ones merely overflow. In time of flood the Ohio moves rapidly only so long
as it is within its channel, drift riding by at what seems to
be packet speed. Thereafter, even while the river rises, it
flattens out. Its so-called tributaries cease to be tribute-
bearers and become tribute-takers. For the time being,
they are bayous. The larger stream sends its overflow water
into them at least as far as the first riffle, farther if there is
a real flood. Sometimes it throws its tributaries into pools
for forty or fifty miles. At such times, little rivers which
run almost dry in summer would be navigable by steamboats and flatboats, and in the old days these boats were
upon them.

The water which backs up into Cincinnati's streets is
slow water, and that is a saving fact. In the usual flood,
which comes in the late winter or early spring every two
or three years, the river rises from pool stage of nine feet
to flood stage of fifty-two feet and goes on to about sixty
feet. But the flood which swept in near the end of January,
1937, was not the usual flood. It was twenty feet higher
than that, putting the waterworks and the power-and-light
plant out of commission, overturning gasoline tanks in the
industrial area along Mill Creek, and starting fires which
threatened a general conflagration.

Had Cincinnati been a town of the Middle Ages, life,
outside the inundated area, would have gone on about as
before. The people of that time used tools, not machines;
had no power and needed none save their own hands and
their domestic animals. There were no streetcars or busses,
and no need of them, for the artisan lived above his own
shop. Food came from the surrounding countryside, not
from a distance; and it was the age of wood fires, of candle-
light. Things being as they were, however, our city was as

one in war time. Its streets were half deserted, streetcars were withdrawn from service, factories idle, theaters darkened, schools, shops, and libraries closed, water supply sharply rationed, dwellings as faintly lighted after dark as if a single candle burned in a single window.

Even this extraordinary visitation the city took with a calmness born of its constant preparedness against inundation. But it did one extraordinary thing. Lucius Quinctius Cincinnatus, from whom it took its name, was called from the plow by the people of Rome in a time of grave peril and vested with the rank of dictator—a word which means literally somebody who tells you what to do; in sixteen days he cleaned up, divested himself of his extraordinary powers, and was back between the plow handles. By action of the Council, the Governor and the President, following this ancient pattern in Cincinnati, almost unlimited powers were given the City Manager. "It took the Old Roman sixteen days to mop up," my newspaper said in an editorial at the time. "Perhaps his successor can cut that period in two." He did.

Meanwhile, people on the hilltops lived rather as their grandparents did. Thrown on their own resources they invoked old skills or devices. With little reading possible after nightfall, I learned to play the mouth organ. Lighted candles along the halls of homes illumined a corridor into the past. After the first rush to buy food, housewives discovered that it was wasteful of water to wash dishes; the second rush was to buy paper plates. Then they cast an eye upon the snowbanks in their yards, gathered them in and melted them, though not for table uses. Tubs and boilers were set out to catch rain water which dripped from eaves. Forgotten city springs were remembered again and drawn upon. People with relatives or friends in the country—folk

who drink well water—made pilgrimages to them laden
with jugs and glass jars. It was almost a game to see how
little water the individual could get along with. Coffee or
tea—boiled water, to be sure, but with something else in
it—was drunk instead. Fruit juices had a new vogue. Bathing was out of course and even washing one's face and
hands was a sketchy affair.

Its members are nearly all dead now, but when the
Grand Army of the Republic held its national encamp-
ment in Cincinnati in the summer of 1930, they were still
fairly numerous. One day they went up the river on the
Island Queen to Point Pleasant, and I went along. It was
a memorable occasion. The songs of the nation resounded
from all parts of the boat: "Just Before the Battle,
Mother," "Tramp, Tramp, Tramp, the Boys are Marching," and, above all, "Tenting Tonight on the old Camp
Ground." Under them was the squeal and crash of a veterans' fife-and-drum corps.

Incidents of the river journey were keenly interesting to
people from New England and particularly the West,
where most rivers flow between low banks through a plains
country and only skiffs can navigate them. The amicable
shores in their framework of hills, the numerous bends,
the clear, green water moving easily along at a time when
the flow of other rivers, not locked and dammed, had almost ceased—all were commented upon. Whenever the
boat entered a lock chamber, and mounted to a higher
level, everybody looked over the rail and asked questions.

At Point Pleasant the whole population of the countryside was waiting on the bank. Disembarking, we wound
in a long procession up the hill, through the sycamores
and between corn and tobacco to a plateau. Behind us was
the worn little village, before us the tranquil Ohio.

Through a scene, pastoral and yet masterful, the river flowed from the revelations of one headland to the mystery of the next—a ten-mile straightaway.

What counted with the veterans was that in this little village above Cincinnati was born the man under whom they had marched to victory in a continent-shaking war. The rhythm of those marches beat all unheard in the pulses of the small, plainly dressed, unassuming man who sought service in recruiting offices where gold braid glittered and swords clanked, and the power that slept behind the quiet gray eyes too long remained unguessed. But Grant had had a vision—in his *Memoirs* he admits it—and the march of hosts was in it. The rise of this undramatic country lad to a place where Lincoln could say that he "trusted in God and Grant" is one of America's two great romances. The career of Lincoln, born in the neighboring state of Kentucky—this part of the world was prolific in great men—is the other.

Those river pilgrims are nearly all dead now, and shadows heavier than the river mists overhang that journey to a river shrine. With a tale about Grant's great antagonist I restore it to the archives of memory. The tale has a spectral quality. If the man who told it—a volunteer in the Thirty-ninth Massachusetts—is living now, he is ninety-seven.

Just after Appomattox he saw Lee riding back to his Virginia plantation. For half a mile the young Yankee recruit trudged beside the commander of the vanquished Confederacy. Erect and sad, the Lost Cause, as embodied in the knightly figure of its leader, rode near him, a fellow wayfarer.

"Did Lee speak to you?" I asked.

"Why should he?" was the reply. "I was only a Northern

soldier. His eyes were on the horizon. I don't think he saw me."

"And you didn't venture to speak to him?"

"I would as soon have spoken to a ghost. His eyes haunted me. When I was stationed in Washington I had seen the same sad look on Lincoln's face."

CHAPTER XI

TOWARD THE MOUNTAINS

WE MOVED away from the Public Landing at Cincinnati to the farewell strains of a calliope. There were six score of us aboard and we were headed for the mountains which framed an old American dream, or at least we were headed for Pittsburgh, four hundred and fifty-seven miles up stream. It was a summer night in 1937, and ten o'clock of a Saturday night, which is pretty near a river bedtime. However, people stayed up for a while to watch the lights of the city, and lights of passing towboats reflected in the water. An orchestra was at one end of the long cabin, and some of us took time off for a few dances under the glittering chandeliers of hobnailed glass, always the proper way to begin a steamboat journey. At the other end of the cabin a buffet lunch was set—cheese, crackers, baked beans, hard-boiled eggs, anchovies, coffee. Everybody descended upon it, for there is something in river air which makes you hungry from the start.

The next morning found us lying at Maysville on the Kentucky shore, so that people so minded could attend an early church service ashore—an unfailing steamboat custom which has much to commend it. When we got under way again the traditional routine of a river voyage took shape. This seemed to consist of reading, talking, singing, dancing, and seeking or avoiding the sun or the wind as the vigor of either should indicate. In reality, however, it was something else. We were watching the pictured shores of the river; one girl from Toledo stayed up all night to do so. The forward decks were like a theater gallery commanding a stage where scenes kept shifting.

At awaited intervals came the meals, set at small tables in the cabin, announced by soft-voiced chimes of many tones, served by soft-voiced blacks.

Between these repasts such sight-seeing went on as only a river which rounds another headland every mile or so can afford—a panorama of wooded or pastured hills and bottomlands rich with corn. The wheat harvest was on, and it was the Week of Elderberry Blossoms. Sometimes we went beside shores perfumed like those of Araby the Blest, though with different odors—from the elderberry bloom, from sweet clover, perhaps from mint crushed by the feet of cattle. Songs of birds came from the thickets, among them the voice of the killdeer which sings as it flies—wistful shore songs, all of them. High overhead I saw, or thought I saw, three eagles; they are still to be found along the upper Ohio. At night there were fireflies, and the Summer constellations, low-hanging Scorpio dominant among them, and owl voices by the water's edge.

There was plenty doing on the river itself—the mirrored reflection of willow-bordered shores, cascading torrents flung by the paddle wheels of other craft, silver sheen of water going over the dams. Every little while we met or overtook a towboat carrying coal, sulphur, structural iron, gasoline. Once we had a lively race to reach a lock ahead of four such fleets, becalmed by fog in the lower pool as we had been. The fourth fleet seemed to slow up in sight of the lock to let us pass—"good friends of ours," explained Mrs. Mary Greene, mother of Captain Tom. Twice we slowed up so as not to send a disastrous wash against a fleet of wooden coal boats which were pretty low in the water.

Going around the dams—and we went around about thirty—was a news event. Goods and passengers were taken on and off. Some dog always raced aboard for a call on the cook. A sign told us that the next pool was "normal" and the water in it either rising, falling, or stationary; on our trip it varied from about twelve feet to a fraction over nine. At Montgomery Island, where a high new dam replaces three old ones, the water runs under the wickets instead of over them. When we entered the vast lock chamber and could see naught but the sky overhead, I felt that I was in some audience hall of the Pharaohs.

Farther down on the Kentucky side, we had skirted a county which has that rare thing, a horse theater. I may have blinked when I entered it the year before. What I saw—this was at Germantown—was a roofed amphitheater thronged with more than two thousand spectators. It was two stories high and the posts which supported each floor and ran quite around the arena made it appear as if everybody was sitting in a box. There were more than a hundred such boxes. I thought of the old-fashioned wooden hotels at Saratoga Springs with their spacious courts, on which guests looked down from upper windows. More, however, I thought of the Bowery Theatre and then of the Metropolitan Opera House. Comparison with the latter is made with reservations, for the horse theater is even older than the Metropolitan, with some slight intimation of decrepitude. I sat on bare wood instead of plush, and the interior was whitewashed rather than gilded. For the arena itself, which was two hundred feet wide, the sky was the roof. Except for the track ring it was grassed over. On the inner lawn a few Kentucky colonels were congregated. It seemed to me that this was a Roman amphitheater, although of wood.

Other Kentucky matters came up in boat conversation, including this verbatim report of a Kentucky meal: "Hot biscuits, fried chicken, gravy made with cream; slaw, pickles, new lima beans, hulled October beans cooked long with bacon and hot pepper; squash baked; light mashed potatoes, candied sweets; cream and corn; turnips diced and buttered; tomatoes sliced and stewed; four preserves and jellies; black jam cake, mincemeat pies; coffee, tea, milk, and, best of all, old ham, pan gravy ham sliced in rather short pieces, browned in hot oven in heavy iron skillet, no grease, covered, same time as corn bread."

As we passed a small but lively Kentucky river town one man told how the hotel clerk there sought to interest him by showing him around. On the floor of the barroom was a dark spot. "Blood," explained the clerk. "That's where the barkeeper took a bungstarter and killed a man who was shooting wild." In the town they passed a seemly house with green shutters. "People in there are blind," said the clerk. "Somebody walked in and threw acid on them." Riding in the country, the two passed a barn with a pole and pulley protruding from the eaves by which hay was hauled to the loft. "They hanged a man from that arm last fall," said the clerk.

The strangest tale was that of a Negro soldier, in a World War convalescent camp in South Carolina, who spoke an unknown tongue and had no English. A lettered surgeon discovered that his speech was Highland Scotch (Gaelic). It became a camp game to post the black hillbilly behind a screen and get officers to guessing what he was saying. His story was that he came from a glen in the Kentucky Cumberlands near the Tennessee line where nothing but Gaelic was spoken. The statement seemed incredible, but officers investigated it and found that the sunburnt Scot was telling the truth.

This was the first trip of the *Gordon C. Greene* in its 1937 summer Pittsburgh trade, and therefore something of which the towns along the way took due and friendly notice. A river artist was aboard with the canoe in which he intended to paddle from Pittsburgh back to Cincinnati. Another passenger was a girl from an Arizona ranch who admitted a wish to take a horseback ride through the wildest parts of mountain Kentucky, "where men are men, or think they are." Something of a figure was a veteran born at Moundsville, West Virginia, eighty-five years before. With him the river had been a lifelong passion. He lived in the Iowa town of Shenandoah. For twenty years he tried to get possession of the old *St. Lawrence* whistle, now on another Greene boat. From a Portsmouth engineer he got its double and had it mounted on a Shenandoah laundry, from which it can be heard for six miles away.

From various sources I learned various things. At least one of the twenty-four ocean-going vessels built at Marietta in the preceding century entered the slave trade. On an island two men known respectively as "the Union bully" and "the Rebel bully" of Kentucky's Mason County fought it out with pistols in the Civil War, while both river shores were crowded with spectators; the duel ended the way the war did. Below this point in 1897 was a horse ferry, its treadwheel driven by blind horses; animals that could see would not walk it at all. In high water a floating grocery store and a floating notion store used to enter Cabin Creek in Kentucky and traffic there. Farther upstream, just back of a government lock, is a hamlet called Beavertown, the main industry of which during prohibition was moonshining. After every raid steamboats did a rushing trade bringing up copper washboilers and tubing from Bellaire; once, at high water, these (inferentially) contraband consignments were put off at the government building and passed through to the general store!

Below Steubenville, at the foot of a high hill on the other shore lived the hermit of Brown Island who tended two government lights, spoke to nobody, and was glad when steamboat men tossed him the Pittsburgh papers. As with all hermits, he was supposed to have a hidden hoard. Miscreants broke in upon him, killed him, ripped up the cabin floor—and found nothing.

Enlarging some record of the Ohio's tributaries which I had made elsewhere, on this trip I saw the mouths of the Little Hocking, the Little Kanawha, and the Little Muskingum; the mouth of Yellow Creek, on which the Indian Logan's family was massacred; the mouth of the Beaver, where historic Fort McIntosh was located, and the mouth of the Little Beaver which flows through my natal town, and which has become a river-and-rail terminal.

Captain Greene's mother conducted me on a tour of the lower deck, where I saw roustabouts asleep on cots amid the bales and boxes of the cargo. This included cereals, coffee, soap, kegs of dill pickles, plow handles, oil, automobiles, and frames for overstuffed chairs and sofas. A black dog, a waif of the January floods, kept guard over all this plunder. At Wheeling we took on two carloads of lanterns destined for the Louisville and Memphis markets; the floods had brought a big demand for lanterns in all the river towns. On the way also we loaded seventy tons of coal upon our bow, and after that the steamboat, her nose a little deeper in water, responded more readily to the wheel, and we made eleven miles an hour instead of ten.

At the salt town of Pomeroy the captain told me that until a few years ago he used to freight his boats with its product for the Cincinnati packing houses. His father before him sometimes played both the merchant and the navigator, making a profit—if he was lucky—on the salt as well as on the carrying thereof. This was a common practice with captains taking out Kanawha Valley products. Boats that followed it and brought butter, eggs, and garden truck to the Pittsburgh markets were called huckster boats; I saw the last of these, the *Liberty,* lying dismantled inside the Little Kanawha.

I was entertained by the saga of the little low-water packet, *Cricket,* as confided by its one-time skipper, Captain Hughes, now pilot on our boat. Once it brought fifty thousand hoop poles from the Kanawha forests to East Liverpool to make casks for pottery. When it appeared on the Big Sandy with the first calliope to be heard on those waters, householders and storekeepers deserted their posts and flocked to the banks, and "you could have robbed every place in town." When it carried a hundred tons of ice from Catlettsburg to Pikeville, cold weather set in, the ice froze into a solid mass inside the boat, and it took days to chop it out.

For various other matters a word must suffice: If the air is either ten degrees warmer or colder than the water, there is fog. Marietta has a River Museum. Martin's Ferry, birthplace of William Dean Howells, celebrated its sesquicentennial in 1937. At Ironton is a steamboat warehouse on wheels which can be pulled away from rising water—a Mississippi River device. We saw the cornfield of unforgettable memory, where a packet, traveling blind in fog and high water, settled down for good a furlong back from the river. Mixed railroad trains which carry freight and passengers are "packets" to river men. Every roustabout carries a spoon—not a razor—in his hip pocket.

As we entered the upper reaches of the river, the hills grew even higher, the water was a clear green, and boys swam along shore and waved to the boat. Women passengers waved in return, but only to such boys as wore a little something.

Until about the last sixty miles, the ride up the river is a sort of idyll, something lifted out of the serene American past, and out of a past more serene and more distant, perhaps the age of Theocritus. After that, if you travel the remaining stretch, as we did, through the sunset hour and on to midnight, it is sheer drama, drama that looks ahead. We swept between flaming furnaces under a sky which was stained crimson and gold by that master painter, the Age of Steel.

We passed the point where the two rivers meet to form the Ohio and, creeping up the Monongahela, moored at a wharfboat. At the same moment the *St. Paul* came in beside us from a moonlight excursion, all lights and music and merrymaking. I turned from it to look at the wharfboat lying black and silent. Strange and yet familiar it seemed. This was no mere floating warehouse; it was a dismantled steamboat, largest stern-wheeler that ever plied the rivers, and I had been on it. A whimpering dog was tied on the deck of the old *Queen City*.

CHAPTER XII

CALLING ON THE FRENCH

I WAS sitting on the sea wall at Cairo asking myself what next, when answer came into view on the Mississippi with a band playing and flags flying. The packet swung around into the Ohio, nosed through its swollen current, made port. I went aboard the *Cape Girardeau,* sought its whence and whither, and engaged passage. The questions were mere formalities. What counted was that here was a boat bound for somewhere—a boat I knew nothing about. Mine was a floating vacation. For a fortnight I had been riding various rivers mainly on boats which I knew nothing about. One of the rivers was three hundred feet underground. My conveyances included a big side-wheeler, a small stern-wheeler, a freighter, a launch, a market boat and a dredge boat. Like Malory's knights of the Round Table I was riding at adventure.

I had been lucky thus far, and the luck was holding. The boat which I had boarded was making a Fourth of July week-end run from St. Louis to Cairo and back. In a few hours we were going up the Middle Mississippi.

There are four Mississippis, though boatmen speak of but three. The fourth runs from the Falls of St. Anthony, traditional head of navigation, four hundred and fifteen miles farther up to Leech River, and small steamboats have traveled it. Below it in turn are the Upper River, which is from the Falls to the mouth of the Missouri; the Middle River, which is from the mouth of the Missouri to the mouth of the Ohio, and the Lower River, which is from the mouth of the Ohio to the Gulf. The Middle Mississippi is nearly two hundred miles long. Our boat's course covered all save the final fifteen-mile stretch between St. Louis and the Missouri's mouth.

It was good to find myself again one of a numerous company in holiday mood and attire. After the first night or so of my journey I had had few travel companions, and little conversation except as I made it myself with boatmen, fishermen, shellers, and sundry natives of Indiana, Kentucky, Tennessee, and Missouri. I was rather roughly clad, with no luggage save a haversack, for this was in part a walking trip. All the rivers were high, sometimes I had to walk in mud to get ashore, and the tribute of four states was on my shoes. In the well-dressed throng aboard the packet, however, this made no point of difference. I met friendly people—among them those inveterate summer travelers, a party of schoolteachers—and so far won the favor of the captain that he crowded on steam the second night and arrived at St. Louis ahead of time, which enabled me to catch a train.

Stopping only now and then, we went up the river, Missouri to our left, Illinois to our right. Some places I identified from a chart. I asked questions about others and jotted in my notebook two perhaps inexact statements: that a towhead was a young island, a chute a narrow side river. A number of the names were intriguing. In succession we passed Devils Island, Devils Tea Table, Devils Bake Oven and Devils Backbone. I remember Bee Bluff, Cat Island, Goose Island, Dogtooth Bend, Owl Creek, Turkey Island, Horse Island. Other interesting points were Sawmill Hollow, Pulltight Landing, Isle de Bois Creek, Salt Point, Sycamore Landing, Mud Landing, White Horse, River des Pères, Cabaret Island. Outstanding among young islands was the Belle of Memphis Towhead, formed by the wreck of the steamboat of that name.

Though our packet purchased a breeze, the languors of summer lay upon either shore. July, it seemed, was no month to hold serious debate upon anything. A warm wind blew over the meadows. The wheat harvest was a golden avalanche, or so we guessed. I was minded of a saying in one of Virgil's Georgics that the wild bird homes are red with berries. Over them was the drift of butterflies, and over the fields the hum of glutted bees, the locust's loud loquacities, the jargon of other insects. A hawk stooped from a cloud. Jays in motley sounded in the woods the notes of carnival. A redbird sang one thing, but seemed to be pondering another. With nightfall the river shores became a wailing place for the snipe. Those pioneers in night life, the owl and the bat, emerged. At intervals I heard, or thought I heard, the pleasant sound of cattle cropping grass. There seemed to be an African moon.

So we went along, accepting and appraising the panorama of sky and shore, bestirring ourselves only when the gangplank was lowered. Our first stop was at Cape Girardeau on the Missouri bank fifty miles above Cairo. Though a French town with some historical background, it has another claim on the traveler. Once it was a headland thrusting out into a now-forgotten ocean. All above it was land, all below it was sea; into that sea, and not into the Gulf, the Mississippi poured its burden. Salt water receded, the great river followed, laying down soil as it went, and so built out the continent more than a thousand miles. There are other such capes and peninsulas. Not far below Cape Girardeau the levees begin, and thenceforth the river follows a strange course, running through a groove in a sort of ridge, its surface higher, its bed lower, than land on either side.

This was the first of six old French towns, three on each

side of the river, which we passed on our way upstream. All lie within a stretch of a hundred and forty miles, five in a stretch of seventy miles. The Middle Mississippi is singularly rich in its memorials of French settlement and these towns have a rewarding history. They were settled from Canada and not from New Orleans because the river flows south, expediting navigation in one direction, retarding it in the other, and affording no navigation for fur-laden bateaux except downstream. Half of them were in existence when New Orleans was founded in 1718.

The fur trade brought them into being. In each little town arose a trading post, a fort, a mission. Usually the mission came first, for the zeal and daring of the Jesuit fathers was even greater than that of the voyageurs. Beside the church was a convent, around it whitewashed houses of cross-timbers and clay. Wayside shrines stood along the trails leading to the settlement. Orchards grew up and little farms were tilled, but the main occupation of the villagers was in hunting and trapping on their own account, and buying furs from their wild neighbors. They trafficked with them on distant rivers, and every year the red men paid them a return visit. These were occasions of festivity, for the French understood the savage nature perfectly and—regardless of any ties overseas—strengthened the bond between the two races by taking women whom they called wives, and begetting broods of half-Indian children.

So Kaskaskia, already a village of the Illini, became a French town in 1700, nearly a score of years ahead of New Orleans; it is the oldest permanent settlement in the Mississippi Valley. Cahokia and Fort Chartres became French settlements about the same time as New Orleans. Ste. Genevieve followed in 1735, St. Louis in 1764, Cape Girardeau in 1780. The three on the Missouri side have been under Spanish as well as French rule.

All six have had important moments. St. Louis was once the capital of Upper Louisiana. Fort Chartres was capital of a province of Louisiana. At Cape Girardeau the Spanish established their first government west of the Mississippi in 1793. Kaskaskia was the capital of Illinois Territory. Kaskaskia and Cahokia were seized by George Rogers Clark before he undertook the attack on Vincennes. The river has left Ste. Genevieve two miles inland from its shore. It did worse things to Kaskaskia.

After leaving Cape Girardeau, our boat stopped before Ste. Genevieve. Cars took us back to the town, and we strolled through engaging streets with stucco houses which would not have looked out of place in the French Quarter of New Orleans. The town has a fine old church, a museum, pleasantly redolent memories. The first road west of the Mississippi, called Rue Royale by the French and El Camino Real by the Spanish, ran through it and on to St. Louis in one direction, to New Madrid in the other. Though the country west of the river had been Spanish since 1762, a French officer established a military post in Ste. Genevieve in 1766, for news traveled slowly then, particularly when it had to travel upstream.

Once upon a time a spring flood came upon Ste. Genevieve. The pious villagers urged their priest to "pray away the water" and pledged themselves to share their crops of corn with the church if prayer availed. He waited until the waters had become stationary before he assented to the bargain. Then his prayers floated over them, and slowly they receded, leaving a deposit of fertile soil on the cornland. The villagers had more than an ordinary crop to divide with the church.

When we stopped before one of the French towns—I forget which—the boat's orchestra gave a little concert and people came out on the shore to listen. The captain said that on longer stops the packet sometimes gave a ball and invited villagers aboard to join in the dancing, a survival of what once was called "river bank hospitality." In an earlier day when steamboats stopped at a landing, Negroes would go ashore and carry among the waiting throngs trays laden with fried fish, slices of roast beef, grapes, nuts, tropical fruits, and ices, all with the captain's compliments—which was good salesmanship as well as good fellowship.

A few miles below Cape Girardeau and on the Illinois side we passed two other French settlements without pausing. Fort Chartres, now called Fort Gage, was established in 1720 to protect and promote a mining speculation—gold and lead—in the trans-Mississippi region. To this end, two hundred white men and a larger number of Negro slaves from San Domingo were brought in. The first fort, a wooden stockade, was succeeded in 1753 by a massive stone fortress with walls and bastions two feet thick, pierced with loopholes for muskets and portholes for cannon. An English traveler who saw it in 1766 called it the most commodious fort in the country. But against one enemy it had no defense. Floods destroyed most of it a few years later, and the garrison removed to near-by Kaskaskia. The old powderhouse is still standing and the lower courses of the fort.

Kaskaskia used to lie at the mouth of the Kaskaskia River. That river has two chapters, one representative of the American story, the other as somber and strange a thing as the Great Valley may have known. The waterway is perhaps five hundred feet wide at the mouth, and about five hundred miles long. In high water small steamboats used to ascend it far and bring down corn and wheat. Once it was seven miles longer, and in that vanished reach the somber chapter was written.

Though one enters the Mississippi and the other the Wabash, the Kaskaskia and Embarras rivers head near each other in central Illinois, rather close to the Indiana line. Both have names, one Kickapoo and one French, which troubled the settlers, and were shortened respectively to Okaw and Ambraw. The treeless country between them was called the Grand Prairie. Because the marshlands east of the Embarras confused travelers on the Vincennes Trace, and because the river itself disconcerted them when they followed its course, by sometimes sending its head-waters across to the Wabash instead of downstream to the Mississippi, they gave it a name which means just what it says.

In the upper country served by these small rivers, the tale of pioneer settlement in the meadow lands just west of the Cumberlands was repeated half a century later and largely by men who had come from those meadows on horseback. They found bear and deer, the panther, the wildcat, the timber wolf, the coyote, together with multitudes of wild turkeys, passenger pigeons, paroquets, and prairie chickens. Also they found those common pests of the frontier—rattlesnakes, copperheads, innumerable mosquitos and horseflies; with whisky and native barks and herbs they brewed their own remedies for the afflictions which these things brought upon them.

Along the watercourses grew huge grapevines, berry bushes, and all kinds of oak, nut, and sugar trees. Here was provender for man and beast, and something more. Logs were cut and rolled to the prairie, where they were set up into cabins floored with puncheons, roofed with clapboards, and finished with doors rived from straight-grained, so-called board trees, usually walnut or white oak.

The doors had wooden latches inside, and a latchstring
hanging outside; to lock them, settlers merely pulled in the
string. This was the familiar dwelling of settlers farther
east, with one or two variations. Instead of stones, the outside chimney was of logs coated with clay, and sometimes
fireplaces had backs and jambs of clay-encased sods.

In this rude setting pioneer life wrote a prairie chapter.
Furniture and utensils followed the primitive pattern;
three-legged stools, indestructible chairs with hickory-bark
seats, rag carpets, pewter dishes, wooden piggins, long-
handled gourds, iron skillets, journey boards for baking
corn pone; ash hoppers for making lye and soft soap, spin-
ning wheels, and home-made looms from which came the
coarse woolen and flaxen fabrics that the women fashioned
into garments. The men wore buckskin trousers—thickets
and briars demanded this—and in winter, caps made of rac-
coon, fox or wolfskins. Dances were held in the open air;
corn huskings, spelling bees, and emotional revivals were
after the pioneer tradition, and at all these gatherings
singers followed the so-called buckwheat notes of a song-
book known as *Missouri Harmony*. Such was life a generation before the Civil War on the Second American
Frontier.

Meanwhile the French town of Kaskaskia, seven miles
from the river's mouth on a narrow neck of land between
it and the Mississippi, went its own ways. At first, and long
before there were upstream settlements, these ways were
musical with the chants of nuns and morning and evening
bugle calls from the fort, gay with the uniforms of soldiers,
the kerchiefs of peasant women, the barred eagle feathers
and beaded trappings of vermilion-daubed Indian chiefs.
People lived with little thought of the morrow—which was
rather the custom of Canada-reared French folk. For a
while things went well. "The village of Notre Dame de

Cascasquias," said an English traveler in 1770, "is by far the most considerable settlement in the Country of the Illinois." In 1778 its inhabitants yielded willingly to George Rogers Clark and gave him help in the attack upon Vincennes. In 1812 it became the territorial capital of Illinois. In 1825 Lafayette paid it a visit.

So from time to time did the Mississippi River floods. The first of record was in 1724, when the town was completely submerged. The worst may have been in 1844, when the steamboat *Indiana* carried the nuns and two hundred citizens from Kaskaskia up to St. Louis; for sixty miles the boat navigated the sunken highway, leaving the Mississippi far to the left, and the town itself under twenty feet of water. The citizens came back, but so, a generation later, did the big river, cutting across the cape, seizing the last seven miles of its tributary, and then moving in upon Kaskaskia itself, which had become an island. By 1898 the work was done. When at the end of day our boat swept over the drowned town I looked and listened. By rights, as duly set forth in all legends of sunken cities, I should have seen chancel columns and arches far beneath, and the ruined stalls of a market place, and heard the choiring nuns and the tumults of a ghostly secular traffic floating up through the water. Anyway, I saw a church tower on a new island near the farther shore and heard its bell calling. There Kaskaskia has risen again. Once it had three thousand inhabitants. Now it may have a hundred.

Going on, we saw the noble outlines of the island of Grand Tower, and then a range of bluffs bolder perhaps than any on the Lower River. At journey's end we tied up between two of the six French towns. Cahokia on the Illinois side is now just a name on old maps. Yet there Clark held the most pictorial of all councils with the savage nations of the north; there La Salle found an Indian village in 1682, and beyond the site are vast mounds which carry the tale of continuing settlement into the realm of misty conjecture. St. Louis on the Missouri side is a great modern city, but when you come to it by packet you seem to remember only that it got its start in the raw fur trade and that it had been a jumping-off place for everything west.

CHAPTER XIII

MOONLIGHT BOATS

ON THE Middle Mississippi, somewhat more often than elsewhere, one meets vessels that seem bound for a near-by carnival. They are called moonlight boats. What has come to be known as a moonlight boat and has had other names—for it is as old as history—is a pleasure craft plying upon inland waters. It is neither a packet, a cargo boat, nor a ferry. A packet starts at one place and goes to another more than a day's ride distant; you can sleep upon it, and you do. A cargo boat has also a definite trade and destination; but you cannot sleep upon it, the law forbidding it to carry passengers. A ferryboat makes short trips to and fro across a river, a harbor, or a lake. The moonlight boat simply goes out and comes back the same day. It is without a destination and without sleeping accommodations except for officers and crew. Sometimes it is called a moonlite boat, the bizarre spelling meaning nothing more than that it may make daylight trips as well as those under the moon.

The best authentic account of such a boat is in Plutarch. What it sets forth is the theme of a historical painting, "Embarkation of Cleopatra to Meet Mark Antony," which, a generation or more ago, used to adorn the drop curtains of so-called opera houses in small towns of the Middle West. The scene is a river in Asiatic Turkey, the time about B.C. 41. Antony had summoned Egypt's queen to appear before him and answer the accusation that she had aided Cassius in the wars against him. She took no account of his repeated commands, "and at last, as if in mockery of them (it is perhaps John Dryden's translation) she came sailing up the Cydnus in a barge with gilded stern and outspread sails of purple, while oars of silver beat time to the music of flutes and fifes and harps. . . ."

On this recital Shakespeare based a glowing passage in *Antony and Cleopatra:*

> The barge she sat in, like a burnish'd throne,
> Burn'd on the water: the poop was beaten gold;
> Purple the sails, and so perfumed that
> The winds were love-sick with them; the oars were silver,
> Which to the tune of flutes kept stroke, and made
> The water which they beat to follow faster,
> As amorous of their strokes. For her own person,
> It beggar'd all description: she did lie
> In her pavilion—cloth-of-gold of tissue—
> O'er-picturing that Venus where we see
> The fancy outwork nature: on each side her
> Stood pretty dimpled boys, like smiling Cupids,
> With divers-colour'd fans, whose wind did seem
> To glow the delicate cheeks which they did cool,
> And what they undid did.

Long before that meeting, however, moonlight boats were upon the waters of the world. Though he does not speak of them, one may infer from Herodotus that Babylon knew them, and that when Queen Nitocris had a great lake made above her capital and caused the swift Euphrates to wind so that "the stream might be slacker by reason of the number of curves, and the voyage be rendered circuitous, and that at the end of the voyage it might be necessary to skirt the lake and so make a long round," she had something more in mind than that enemies approaching by water would have to come three times within sight of Babylon before arriving. A city with smooth lake-and-river waters must have had pleasure craft, and the barges of queens who pleasured themselves in hanging gardens would be upon them.

When he speaks of Egypt, the Father of History is more definite, although a trifle reticent. After an account of a king who used captives taken in war to cover the land with a network of canals, so that "it is now unfit for either horse or carriage," and a description of the great lake of Moeris, which he calls "manifestly an artificial excavation," he speaks of a smaller lake in the temple precincts at Saïs: "On this lake the Egyptians represent by night the sufferings of Osiris, and this representation they call their Mysteries. I know well the whole course of the proceedings in these ceremonies, but they shall not pass my lips."

On the lakes and canals of ancient Egypt and on its great river, pleasure craft plied. Of a certain Pharaoh it is recited that in the pond in his garden he had a boat "manned by twenty women with the most beautiful breasts and backs, none of whom had ever borne a child; their oars were of ebony and gold, the handles encrusted with gold and silver." At one point, twenty nets were cast over the women, while a wooden mummy was carried about in a coffin and a slave-poet sang to them. Cleopatra must have known of this. Of course she had taken part in the immemorial Nile Festival, celebrated every year on a summer night, to mark the fructifying embrace of the swollen river and panting land—and never more madly than under later Arab rule when the waterway was alive with lanterned boats and women danced on illuminated barges while spectator throngs indulged the license of carnival.

One catches glimpses in books of other moonlight fleets: the barge of Haroun-al-Raschid in the *Thousand and One*

Nights, slipping silently through the dark along the canals
of Bagdad while with his own eyes and ears the caliph
learns what his subjects are about; scenes in Chinese cities,
where innumerable thousands dwell in houseboats on
rivers or on the Grand Canal, and under the dramas of
life and love and death there is quiet or flowing water;
the boats that ply the flower-bordered lakes and canals surrounding the City of Mexico.

But here I would speak only of what I know at first
hand, dismissing all adventures of others with a passing
note of regret that when I was in Nippon two years ago,
I was unable to accept the invitation of a Japanese friend
and spend an evening in his company on the canals of
Tokyo, with a group of blossom-faced samisen-plucking
geishas to entertain us.

I did, however, have a daylight ride in a great canoe—
and in good company—down a wild river of Japan. Our
course was between steep mountain walls clothed with
cypress trees in which monkeys clambered, and under
which rhododendrons, camellias, and azaleas wrought the
pageantry of Maytime. At the end of that journey there
was tea in a waterside villa where eight celebrated Japanese
poets, who had been before us, had hung their verses on
its walls.

In our own country the moonlight boats perform a
kindred service of sentiment, satisfying in some measure a
perhaps unconscious wistfulness in the life of river towns
since the fading of the Steamboat Age. They are to be
found, though it be only as illuminated flats under tow, on
the deeper reaches of streams which have long been closed
to navigation. Hundreds of towns are children of the inland waters. A generation or so ago their activities were
attuned to the clangor of the side-wheelers. Now they are

not content to forget altogether the element that brought them forth. Though few of their inhabitants have ever ridden on a packet, nearly all have taken afternoon and evening trips on excursion boats, some of them former packets whose staterooms have been ripped out. The towns may be hot in midsummer, but there is always a breeze on the river, and sunset and moonrise, and the satisfying sounds of sighing smokestacks and lapping water. So for brief intervals these communities reaffirm their ancient loyalties.

All up and down the rivers the annual coming of the moonlight boats is awaited. Advance posters with gaudy lithographs set the dates, and schools, lodges, political groups, and family parties engage passage. When I went up the Ohio to Pittsburgh, I saw the *St. Paul*—a St. Louis boat—just pulling out of the Monongahela wharf where we made fast. When I went down the Ohio to Louisville I saw the *Idlewild* carrying away a throng of picknickers. When I went up the Mississippi to St. Paul, I found another boat, the *Capitol,* at our wharf and boarded her for a midnight ride.

The major ports of the excursion craft are Pittsburgh, Cincinnati, Louisville, St. Louis, St. Paul, and New Orleans. Five of these cities have daily service in summer, one of them, New Orleans, throughout the winter. In both spring and fall the boats make trips to the smaller towns. Their main range is the Mississippi, and most of them operate out of St. Louis, chief excursion port of the country. At various places along the river I have seen the St. Louis boats. Their up-river itineraries include such towns as Hannibal, Quincy, Keokuk, Burlington, Davenport, Dubuque, Prairie du Chien, La Crosse, Winona, and Red Wing. Down river, they stop at Cape Girardeau, Cairo, Memphis, Helena, Friars Point, Arkansas City, Greenville,

Vicksburg, Natchez, Baton Rouge, and a few smaller ports. The *Island Queen* of Cincinnati also roves the rivers in spring and autumn.

It takes two crews and a total of a hundred or more persons to man one of the boats. These include officers, pilots, engineers, firemen, watchmen, deck hands, cooks, maids, waiters, musicians, clerks, cashiers, dance floor monitors, ticket sellers. The men who operate the boats have staterooms and living quarters in the texas. When there are long stops at the cities, the others live ashore at their homes or in family hotels and boardinghouses.

These excursion boats are the largest and showiest of all craft on the rivers. They are very wide, they are longer than the average city block, and they have five or more decks. Their dancing floors are expertly made, the orchestras competent. White without, their interiors—walls, booths, stair rails, and counters—are in vivid harmonies of green, orange, and red. With their flags flying, their calliopes clamoring, and deck upon deck ablaze with lights which are repeated in the river, they lay a spell on the night and on the water.

Nearly three thousand or more persons can be accommodated on any one of them. A mere thousand are almost lost in its wide spaces. The largest of them, the new *Admiral,* which I saw lying in port at St. Louis, can carry five thousand persons. Built all of steel, streamlined and aircooled, it made me think at once of a battleship, the most modern type of streetcars, and the fast railroad trains which I had seen speeding along both banks of the Upper Mississippi.

My moonlight ride out of St. Paul—I have had such rides out of other cities—was on a sister boat, which lay so near our packet that I could almost step from one to the other. Roy Streckfus, master of the *Capitol,* and "Buck" Leyhe, master of our *Golden Eagle,* were friends of long standing, and the river has a courteous tradition. On another trip the packet tied up beside a showboat, which had everybody come aboard for its performance. On this trip we were invited to join some thousands of Minnesota folk and be guests for the evening of Captain Roy. We all accepted.

As slowly the excursion boat drew out from the dock and headed down the river, its calliope whooped farewells and hundreds of cars answered with their horns. In procession they followed us for some miles along the left bank. We went through a drawbridge, past the odorous stockyards zone, beside lighted houseboats that in the river's mirror seemed of many stories, and then left the city behind and moved on between shadowy shores, nor turned back until we reached a dam fifteen miles below. A lopsided moon had swung up. Out of the hot night came a cool wind. There was a good black orchestra, and most of our contingent danced. It was midnight when we trooped across to the packet, some to don pajamas and sit for a while on the hurricane deck in hope that the wind would come upstream.

CHAPTER XIV

THE UPPER MISSISSIPPI

I WENT aboard the *Golden Eagle* on a mid-July midafternoon. This was at St. Louis in 1940. The waterfront attracted me. There was the wharf-boat, long and low, with a dim interior charged with re-membered odors of fruits, salt meat, and salt fish, and thronged with black-skinned roustabouts—one of the few wharfboats left on inland waters. Near it lay the showboat *Goldenrod*, a sign announcing that *Adrift in a Great City* was playing there. Back of the two boats was a paved and sloping levee, and beyond it a row of ancient brick build-ings. This was authentic river stuff, of about the period of Grover Cleveland's first administration.

The waterfront attracted me still more than St. Louis itself. It is a big and rather beautiful city, with a noticeable skyline; but people who travel the rivers, though they have quite a liking for towns, take big cities for granted. When they get to the top of the Hill, as they call the river bank, their curiosity may be exhausted. Along the entire navi-gable length of the Mississippi, which is more than two thousand miles, there is only one exception to this. That is New Orleans which, from the very beginning, held forth its arms out of the Deep South with such a gesture of be-guilement toward the cruder folk of the Northern settle-ments that it might almost be said the American flatboat, keelboat, broadhorn, and steamboat were invented in order to avail of the invitation. In this sense the Creole capital created the navigation of the Mississippi.

There was a little something to be said, however, for our

port of embarkation that was more in the line of our peculiar interests, and this I found in a government document. St. Louis is the world's greatest market for mules and furs. Mules and furs—and small towns—all are primitive things, like flowing water itself, and therefore within the scope of one's understanding and sympathies. With a friendly backward glance I walked through the wharfboat, up the gangplank to the main deck of the packet, and thence up a flight of stairs to the purser's office. There quarters were assigned me, a black porter carrying my baggage up another flight of stairs which led from the misnamed boiler deck to the well-named hurricane roof. My stateroom was in the rear of the texas, which rose from this roof, and so near was the room to the stern wheel that its plashings lulled my slumbers during the thirteen hundred miles of river travel that lay ahead.

Besides an upper and lower bunk, the room had lifebelts, two chairs, a corner stand with towels, soap, and a basin and pitcher of water—and space enough to turn around in. It looked snug. I liked it.

My first chore was to make a tour of the boat. What I learned then was eked out later by fragmentary conversations with its master, Captain W. H. "Buck" Leyhe, who is bluff and friendly but about as tight-lipped as the mussel shells, miscalled "clams," which are the basis of an important river industry. He is quoted as declaring that he had read but one book in his life. Although a certain book of mine devoted four chapters to an account of a journey I had in another boat with him as its master, that was not the book he read; but he was good enough to say he had heard of it. The captain is tall, burly, and hearty, with a voice that would split a gale endwise. He likes to play poker with other officers and with passengers; he seems to win only now and then.

For his boat there grew up in me and in my shipmates the affection one has for small, competent objects. The *Golden Eagle* had less tonnage than the first steamboat that went down the Mississippi. It was only one hundred and eighty-five feet long, or, counting the wheel, perhaps two hundred and ten feet overall. At the beginning of our voyage it drew but four and one-half feet of water. Toward the end when its heaping coal bunkers were nearly empty, and two pyramids of watermelons had disappeared in table onslaughts, it drew just four feet. In high water, save for snags and floodgates, it could have navigated most of the creeks of the Republic.

When we stopped for half an hour at the Iowa town of Clinton so that a woman passenger could call on a friend there—the captain is good-natured to a fault, as the saying goes—I studied his boat from the shore, and made the mental note that it looked like a bull pen, a haymow, a caboose, and the Siege of Vicksburg all rolled into one. Yet the little stern-wheeler rode the waves easily and carried its years lightly—it was built as a cotton packet at New Orleans in 1907 and rebuilt some years later—and, believe it or not, it has been officially acclaimed as the fastest steamboat on our rivers; this despite the captain's realistic and humorous dissent that it was "just a ten-mile boat."

It won its deer-horn pennant in 1939, he admitted, by racing against time—which meant riding down the swollen Mississippi in competition with two California boats that had to buck the tide on their trips down the San Joaquin and Sacramento rivers to the Pageant of the Pacific. The winner made one hundred and twenty-eight miles at the rate of 13.8 miles an hour, three miles better than either rival's record.

Though I was already hungry when we set forth—that is

what the mere thought of river travel is apt to do to you —it wanted three hours to dinner. After looking over the boat I used the remainder of the time in looking over the passengers. The packet was almost crowded. It will carry ninety-four first class, and I counted eighty-five fellow passengers, somewhat more than half of them female, as older boat lists would have put it. The proportion of young men and young women was larger than in any of my previous river trips; several of the girls were quite pretty, some more than that. My favorite, however, was perhaps a little old lady from St. Louis, with two sumptuous daughters aboard, a streak of amiable cussedness, a conviction that young hussies would be going bare-naked next year or soon thereafter, and two memories of Cincinnati—"the spider-legged cars that go up Mt. Adams," and "that water that runs through the town, and does it still run?" By this she meant the old canal.

Passengers came from nine states, nearly all Midwestern folk—Ohio, Indiana, Illinois, Michigan, Missouri—but with a few from Massachusetts, Oklahoma, Louisiana, and the nation's capital. Among them were devotees of river travel who had gone everywhere that Eagle Packet boats would take them and were making return trips. These included former steamboat officials, ex-pilots with their wives and children. The great-grandfather of one young man had made a fortune in lead at Galena (which is the Latin word for lead) and then put his money in packets of which he bought or built twenty-two; he sold out and engaged in another big river industry, the cutting, rafting, and milling of lumber from the white pine forests of the Mississippi's northern tributaries.

Others aboard included an artist, a physician, a patent lawyer, a hardware merchant, a philatelist, several schoolteachers, a number of office girls. Getting down to names, among the passengers were Captain Sam Smith, St. Louis editor; John Fox of the far South, who has had a good deal to do with the return of the Upper Mississippi to startlingly beautiful life after a quarter century of neglect; for a top card, the grandmother of Ducky Medwick's young wife, a smart old lady whose verses won a steamboat prize. One other shipmate must be noted. With confused recollections of "Tugboat Annie," people aboard got to calling her Towboat Mabel, though she was quite another sort of person—a joyous, tireless young brunette who writes up-river news for the *Waterways Journal*. She knows everybody on the Mississippi, and towboat captains blow their whistles when they pass the pearl-button town of Muscatine, which is her Iowa home.

All in all, the boat with its boatload was a miniature copy of the country, not as of the moment but as of a time that seems to have been fairer. "So we went loafing down the river," said Huckleberry Finn. The *Golden Eagle* went loafing up the river, at about a ten-mile gait, its passengers easygoing, unassuming, comfortable, rather talkative folk. Strangers surveyed one another with eyes of casual friendliness, and after the first meal there were next to no strangers aboard.

Here is a sample introduction:

"Hello!"

"Hello also!"

"What's your name?"

"I am Dosia."

"And what else?"

"You wouldn't remember anyway."

And that, as a certain cartoonist would say, was the Beginning of a Beautiful Friendship, only slightly crimped when later the man in the case led the lady out on the cabin floor, and discovered that as a dancing teacher she was wont to put all men through their paces.

This brings me up to meals. The cabin was too narrow to eat in. Dancing up and down that long narrow passage with its white panels and glittering chandeliers was like dancing from end to end of one of those old Southern mansions which have a hall running clear through them. So passengers ate on deck at dinner and at every meal thereafter, performing this pleasant but intimate social function in sight of people on both shores all the way to St. Paul and back. Long tables were set in the bow, smaller ones on both sides. My own was on the port side, which meant that I had the evening sun for dinner. When it dazzled, strips of canvas were pegged up.

There was fried chicken and a good soup for our first meal, like every meal that followed well cooked and served. In some respects the packet became a floating chapter of the Old South, the veritable South of magnolia blossoms and moonlight. The Negro help made it so. If I say that their manners were more urbane than those of the white crew, in whom was the bluff heartiness of the West, I need to add that their manners were also a shade better than those of the white passengers. They seemed to carry on the tradition of servants in the "big house" of ante-bellum days. Wearing spotless jackets, greeting persons at their own tables with a flashing smile of welcome, serving them promptly and noiselessly, anticipating their wants, the black waiters transformed every meal into something like a social function. The maids were comely creatures, eager to please, knowing how, and so dependable that few passengers locked their staterooms when they were on deck. All these women took a lively personal interest in the travelers whose quarters they looked after. When night came, they doffed their blue dresses, put on white, and from the darkened outskirts of the crowd, listened to the concerts, watched the merrymaking, and complimented their special charges on their singing or dancing.

I remember the first meal, as the scene of the only accident, if you can call it that, of our voyage. I had been watching the river with its low green shores and brown water reaches, and scanning the western bank so I might see where the Missouri came in—the end of any river being to me an occasion of satisfactory solemnity. At last its broad mouth came into view with a turbid current pouring from it. I hoped we would not pass too quickly; nor did we. There was a sudden shock. The packet quivered, came to a stop, and lay motionless for more than half an hour in full sight of the Missouri gateway. Nobody knew what was wrong. I guessed that a log, what on the Ohio is called a "hull inspector," had done an untoward thing to our paddles and marveled at the placidity of other diners.

Later I asked the captain. He said the pilot had steered a little "high"—whatever that is—and grounded the boat on a sand bar. This conversation was at Alton where we went through the first of twenty-six locks on the Upper River, the boat rising a dozen feet to the next pool. All the passengers were on the upper deck watching. As at the other locks, spectators lined the walls, some of them to greet friends aboard. We saw them from two levels, at first from far enough below to note how short are the dresses of the moment, and again, as the lock chamber filled with swirling water, to appraise the quaint pattern of any woman's hat when you look down upon it.

In this neighborhood, on the noble Piasa bluffs, I studied what, until quarrymen destroyed it, was perhaps the most interesting object on the continent. Joliet and Marquette in 1673 saw two dragon forms painted on the cliffs, on which no Indian dared look long. Each (says Père Marquette) was "as large as a calf, with horns on the head like a deer, a fearful look, red eyes, bearded like a tiger, the face somewhat like a man's, the body covered with scales, and the tail so long that it twice makes a turn of the body passing over the head and down between the legs, and ending at last in a fish's tail." Here is evidence that the Dragon Myth, the most profound of all creations of the dreaming mind of man, was in the New World as well as in the Old.

CHAPTER XV

THEY LIVED BESIDE IT

IN THE dusk, not long after leaving Alton, Illinois, on the opening night of our trip up the Mississippi from St. Louis to St. Paul, we passed the mouth of the second of the great river tributaries whose story had always intrigued me. This was the Illinois. It is five hundred miles long. Its mouth, where it comes in at Grafton, is about as wide as the Ohio at Cincinnati; it is navigable with its canal connections clear to the Great Lakes at the port of Chicago, and over it in the last year of record more than six hundred steamboat trips, more than four thousand barge trips, were taken, tonnage representing values in excess of a hundred million dollars.

Yet this waterway seems to be little remarked, perhaps because most large rivers either draw the boundaries of states or drain a number of them. The Illinois draws no boundaries save those of counties, and beginning and ending in one state is by that token a private domain, with some quality of seclusion. But I happen to know it. Laid end to end with the Mississippi, the two of them are about as long as the Missouri. Oddly enough, steamboats were on the latter before they were on the Upper Mississippi, the Lower and Upper Rapids (Des Moines and Rock Island) presenting an impediment to navigation until canals were built around them.

Between the lower stretch of the Illinois and the Mississippi is Calhoun County, one of the few in the Middle West without a railroad, the two bordering rivers providing haulage for its goods. It is shaped like a banana but ought to be shaped like an apple, for its orchards are so vast and so burdened in the fall that their cider is piped into tankers like those for oil, and taken down river to the vinegar factories of Alton.

Above this apple province is one Pike County. Across the Mississippi in Missouri is another. We passed between them in the night. John Hay's *Pike County Ballads* has given them a place in American letters. He says he meant both of them. As he puts it, "The people of the two Pike Counties are very much alike, and they have a dialect speech, a point of view and an intellectual attitude in common. I have encountered nothing else like it anywhere." Those points are paraded in six poems written when Hay was a young man. The inspiration came in church on a hot summer Sunday when a Pike County parson who hadn't a trait of humorous perception in his make-up, droned out a story substantially the same as that in "Little Breeches."

"As I sat there in the sleepy sultriness of the summer," Hay continues, "I fell to thinking of Pike County methods of thought, of what humor a Pike County dialect telling of the story would have, and of what impression the story itself, as solemnly related by the preacher, would make upon the Pike County mind." On the train to New York he wrote "Little Breeches." The lilt and swing of a regional balladry took sudden but transitory hold of him. In one week he wrote the six numbers. Then, as he says, "There were no more Pike County ballads in me, and there never have been any since." His slender collection made a stir. Phrases from it were on every tongue. Critics saw in it a new and valid literary form.

Two of the six are likely always to be remembered. "Little Breeches" tells the story of a four-year-old boy who

"chawed terbacker jest to keep his milk-teeth white." Lost
on the prairie in a wild snowstorm, he was found by his
father, safe and warm among the lambs in a sheepfold.
"How did he git thar? Angels." The rustic sire concludes
that "saving a little child . . . is a derned sight better business than loafing around the Throne." The other memorable ballad tells of Jim Bludso, engineer of the *Prairie
Belle,* who "had one wife in Natchez-under-the-Hill, and
another one here in Pike." When fire broke out on his
crazy old packet, he did, as he swore he would:

> "I'll hold her nozzle agin the bank
> Till the last galoot's ashore,"

and died in doing it.

Hay brought the various Pike Counties into national
consciousness. There are ten of them, all—according to
legend—the abodes of primitive Americans who spend
much of their lives in 'coon hunting, esteem snake oil as
a medicine, grow more than their share of sorghum, and
contend that their log cabins are better ventilated than
other dwellings. Of Missouri's Pike County two conflict-
ing reports arose in the Far West: one that its first migrants were a vagabond folk, "pikers," that is to say okies
of a preceding century; the other that the word was once
a term of honor because people from there paid their
debts, and that sharpers brought it into disrepute by claim-
ing to hail from Pike County.

I slept well the first night, breakfasted late, and then
mingled with fellow travelers. Women were knitting and
gossiping. Men and women were playing poker, rummy,
bunco—tough names, perhaps, yet innocent pastimes. People were reading river books. Down in the cocktail lounge,

if interested, you could hear reports over the air from the Chicago Democratic Convention; and this reminded me that a dozen years before, while riding on a still smaller packet, up the Green River in Kentucky, I had heard the Houston Convention place Al Smith in nomination. On the hurricane deck young women were taking their first sun baths, their skirts pulled well above bare knees, but not half so high as on the nine days that followed, when the Scourge of Heat descended on the continent.

For myself, I watched the river. I had heard that its current cleared above the Missouri, but it still ran brown water, which, however, was less burdened with silt. It was broader than the Lower Mississippi. This meant that it was shallower, its volume much less than farther down, after the Illinois, Missouri, Ohio, Arkansas and Red—major rivers, all of them—had entered it. I soon remarked the number of great blue herons that haunted it. They were nearly always in sight, standing stiltlike on the banks, perched on the upper limbs of toppling sycamores, threading narrow, canal-like streets of water, winging across wide reaches with a heavy assured flight as of freighted argosies. With their heads drawn in against their shoulders and their long legs stretched straight behind them, their goings and comings added an almost archaic touch to the traffic of the river.

They seemed to be border patroons, and with some sort of geographical function, and I myself to be upon a geographical mission following a long boundary line, which set metes and limits to ten states of the Republic. There arose the memory of old school geographies. That was Missouri on the right bank, Illinois on the left (such directions always assume that the traveler is coming down the river); other states were to follow. I was unrolling an

old map and trying to recall physical contours and principal industries of states as I had known them. The river
cities that lay ahead—Quincy, Keokuk, Burlington, Davenport, Rock Island, Dubuque—I could recall various items
about them in the newspapers. I was drawn toward Keokuk, and for a ridiculous reason. In an opera club which
put on Victor Herbert's *Mademoiselle Modiste,* I had
taken part in a chorus beginning:

> Our Culture Club in Keokuk,
> If you belonged you'd be in luck,
> Our meetings are exclusive and delightful!

We reached the Missouri town of Hannibal during the
morning and found busses waiting which took us through
Mark Twain Land. That was the only place along the
Upper Mississippi where getting from the water front into
the town was not a problem. Elsewhere were no streetcar
connections, no busses, no taxis, no telephones. Davenport
has a spacious and sightly public landing, and St. Paul
a small one with some slight sculptural quality. But usually we made fast amid horseweeds and ragweeds, or at
the foot of straggling unpaved trails which angled up the
benches to the city level. The shore communities, most
of them, have turned their backs on the Great River which
begat them, and almost ignore it.

Instead of the Father of Waters, as the Algonquins
christened it, let us call the Mississippi the Forgotten
River. A year ago a new river took its place, of which few
seem to have heard. It is of almost incredible loveliness.

Hannibal has a population of twenty thousand, and
cement works, a limekiln, a large shoe factory; but it is
known to the outside world only as Mark Twain's boyhood home and the scene of youthful adventures recorded

in *Tom Sawyer* and *Huckleberry Finn.* I saw the small
house where he lived, every room of it familiar, for a
movie of some years back was filmed on the spot. Aunt
Polly's bedroom, the home of Becky Thatcher, the Cave,
the poetic statue of Tom and Huck on some lark together,
all are items of tourist interest. In a park far above the
town, and commanding a great sweep of the Illinois bot-
toms, is a bronze statue of the author who made Hannibal
a place of pilgrimage. It pictures him as I remember
seeing him a few years before his death, with flowing hair
and mustache, but without an overcoat. Wearing the overcoat, and gazing out upon the river with a stern watchful-
ness, he looked rather like a politician of practical bent
but responsible quality. On the pedestal was the statement,
"His religion was humanity."

Twain's life was perhaps a demonstration of a statement, I think by Chesterton, that an author's richest materials are the harvest of his boyhood experiences. When he
got too far away from home his first fruits were *Innocents
Abroad,* once a humorous classic, but to modern eyes the
self-portrait of a raw young Middle Westerner deriding
what he could not understand. *Roughing It,* laid in the
Far West, is far better, for in the crude mining country
the author was at home.

His fame rests securely on two river works: *Life on the
Mississippi,* which is a travel book, and the novel, *Huckleberry Finn.* In both the vigorous, joyous, reckless sky-
larking and extravagantly braggart spirit of a great interior
region not long past the frontier era finds perhaps an
ultimate expression. The novel has been called America's
greatest, and I am not disposed to challenge the judg-
ment. Satisfying and utterly beguiling is its narrative of
the runaway lad, drifting down the Mississippi on a raft

with two uninvited hobo guests, one calling himself the "Duke of Bridgewater," the other professing to be "the long-lost Dauphin," both collaborating in staging rap-scallion shows at the river towns. Like the Odyssey, *Huckle-berry Finn* is a Wandering, and out of wanderings the best works of fiction are wrought. That Twain's work, like Homer's, takes its characters on a voyage, and has them perform strange feats and encounter strange folk ashore, is another and a noteworthy parallel.

About bedtime on the second night of our own quiet odyssey, I saw a dim glimmer on the hills upon the Illinois side. This was Nauvoo. It may have nine hundred in-habitants. There was a time when it had fifteen thousand, and was the best-looking and best-managed town in Illi-nois, with a handsome temple, wide thoroughfares, smart shops. Joseph Smith, founder of the Mormon faith, made it so. A poor white of the Yankee breed, but with the blood of ecstatic Puritanism in his veins, he began life as a well digger in upstate New York, and by logical degrees became a gold digger in a region where people believed that the Senecas were descendants of the Ten Lost Tribes of Israel.

It was natural that he should discover, or profess to dis-cover, a volume of golden leaves, and the magical Biblical spectacles, "Urim and Thummim," by which he could translate it. This became the *Book of Mormon,* based on the contention that the Lost Tribes had come to America and were a part of its aboriginal population; strange cir-cumstance it is that when the Mormons were driven out of Nauvoo and trekked west across the Great Plains to Utah, they alone, among all the emigrants, were treated with uniform kindness by the Indians.

Smith had so-called visions, one of them ordaining

polygamy, some of them far-sighted. On Christmas Day in 1832 he made a prophecy which began: "Verily thus sayeth the Lord concerning the wars that shall shortly come to pass, beginning at the rebellion of South Carolina . . For behold the Southern States shall be divided against the Northern States, then the Southern States shall call on other nations, even the nation of Great Britain." Among other things, Joseph Smith prophesied his own death. It came at the hands of a mob in June, 1844, and the exodus to Utah followed.

Though religious and moral motives were avowed by the rioters, the thing that set them marching was what set the borderers of southwestern Pennsylvania marching against the Moravian settlements in eastern Ohio during the Revolution: the spectacle of societies more prosperous and civilized than their own. Smith's followers were dull-witted folk, but his own executive gifts—for he was a great man—and his use of tithes and co-operation gave Nauvoo advantages over neighbor communities. So mobs killed him and ran his followers out, and now Nauvoo is a dim light on the hills and has perhaps nine hundred inhabitants.

I close this chapter with the more edifying tale of another noted American who once commanded a river fort farther north, and who was feted rather than mobbed by a river town farther south where he lived. Aboard our boat I came across a colorful bit of history which carried back by a chain of living men almost a century, fetching up at the Louisiana cotton plantation of a President of the United States, who was also father-in-law of the future President of the Confederate States. Captain Buck told it as he had it from Captain S. T. Waddlington, pilot on the Middle Mississippi, who had it in turn from Captain J. P.

Drouillard, pilot on the steamboat *J. M. White* which was then in the St. Louis-New Orleans trade. When that boat reached Baton Rouge in January 1849, Drouillard saw an up-bound packet, loud with bands and gay with flags, waiting there to take Zachary Taylor, popular hero of the Mexican War, on his way to Washington and the White House. This was all he could remember.

His slight sketch may be filled in from other sources. In procession the people of Baton Rouge escorted the President-elect aboard his boat. There he received a call from Henry Clay, who was coming down river on a trip to New Orleans: the Whig leader was Taylor's picture of a great statesman, and his own wife had prayed that the party might nominate the Kentuckian instead of Old Rough and Ready. Proceeding upstream, the general's boat turned off the Mississippi at Cairo, came up the Ohio, and stopped at Cincinnati where a grand ball was given in his honor. Pretty women hugged and kissed him, as indeed women had at other stops on both rivers. Thus may have begun an American custom which has never been suffered to lapse—exercise of an assumed right of young women to collect gallant salutations from Old Heroes for their memory chests. None of the heroes ever protested.

CHAPTER XVI

PADDLE WHEELS

DAY by day the commerce of the river moved before the eyes of passengers on the *Golden Eagle* as it paddled northward toward St. Paul. Ours was the only packet upon it, but often boats of other kinds hove into view. Showiest of these were the moonlight excursion boats. The sober work of the Mississippi was carried on by small, powerful, snub-nosed towboats pushing barges filled with grain that was poured into them from riverside elevators which somehow looked like a child's toy-house but were bigger. A single tow would hold as much as six loaded freight trains, and maximum tows may have more than a score of barges and a length of one thousand two hundred feet, which compares with that of de luxe liners on the Atlantic.

Quietly, without blast of whistles or other fanfare, the towboats are doing a carrying trade beyond the capacity of whole squadrons of the vanished packets. The timbers of the latter lie here and there in weedy boat yards, their bells and whistles have been salvaged for other craft, and now and then you see what was once a pilothouse doing shore duty as a pavilion on some lawn overlooking the river. When the railroad, pushing westward, reached the Mississippi, its shriller whistle foredoomed the older type of river craft. The completeness of their disappearance was as amazing as the fullness of their heyday.

In 1852 there were three thousand steamboat arrivals at St. Louis; in 1862 more than a thousand at St. Paul. In 1857 two dozen steamboats lay at one time at the

St. Paul levee. About the same year the total steam tonnage on the Mississippi and its tributaries was claimed to be larger than the total steam tonnage of Great Britain upon the high seas. Now little but the names of the thronging river fleets of yesterday remain and you have to go to books to learn them. Five, at least, had names suggesting our own craft: *Little Eagle, Flying Eagle, Spread Eagle, Gray Eagle, War Eagle.* Other names were set forth in rhyming array in an old river song, among them *Golden Gate* and *Sucker State; Helen Mar* and *North Star; Pauline, Kate Keen,* and *Josephine; Wild Boy* and *St. Croix; Gazelle* and *Mountain Belle.* Another group of steamboat names was astronomical, these including *North Star, Saturn, Satellite, Silver Crescent, Eclipse, Equator,* and *Time and Tide.* In still others, like *Volunteer, Lumberman, Last Chance, Monitor, Brother Jonathan, Smelter,* and *Cyclone,* the activities and idiom of the frontier were reflected.

Among random items of river history I was told that Chief Winneshiek is buried with his horse on an Iowa bluff overlooking the river. The legends of Prairie du Chien speak of a French woman who had a dozen husbands and lived to be a hundred and one years old, and of an early citizen who was the first millionaire in all the West. The original Pike's Peak is in Iowa near the town of McGregor and not in Colorado. It is five hundred and forty feet above the Mississippi. The soldier-explorer, Zebulon M. Pike, climbed and named both peaks, the taller one a year after the other. Sentinel Ridge in Wisconsin was the cemetery of some vanished race, whose dead look down on the Mississippi from mounds nearly six hundred feet above.

I learned that because of the two great rapids—now

drowned by dams—packets on the Upper Mississippi were always smaller than those on the Lower; before canals were built around the rapids, keelboats were used at times to help steamboats through them. On the early wood-burning packets passengers went ashore and rambled about while billets were taken aboard, which was once every three hours. Instead of staterooms there were two tiers of bunks on each side of the long cabin, and these were curtained off at night—a device borrowed from the canal boats and loaned to the Pullmans. Whenever boats changed owners, they changed names; some have had as many names as chronic divorcees.

Setting down other scattered items, fogs are rarer on the Upper Mississippi than on the Ohio. There are two hundred and sixteen islands with names, others known only by numbers. There are sixty-two sloughs and twenty-three towheads. There are twenty-four vehicular bridges between St. Louis and St. Paul. There are three hundred and fifty-nine crossing lights to steer by between St. Paul and Cairo. Away from the steering wheel—so the captains aver—pilots are accounted a dumb generation; yet in 1884 the British Government engaged four of them from the upper river to steer boats along the Nile on the military expedition for relief of Chinese Gordon at Khartoum.

On the way upstream I saw a number of dead fish floating on the surface, and I wondered. Then we came upon a suction dredgeboat, which was at work above a hidden bar and discharging sand, gravel, and turbid water on a spoil bank through a long pipe line laid over a fleet of pontoons; when fish emerged, their story was told. Dredging by suction or by dippers or by clamshell buckets goes on somewhere all the time upon every navigable river. Wherever a tributary comes in, bars form. After high water there is always shoaling, usually on a bend or just below or above it, or at the head or foot of islands. Islands are notorious bar-breeders, because the narrow back-channel is sometimes shorter than the other, and water travels faster through it, forming an eddy that deposits sand where it meets the main channel.

Sluggish, winding channels behind islands perform a present service and have a singular historical background. They are called sloughs. In them boats lie up when winter prisons the Mississippi under a sheet of ice perhaps as far down as St. Louis. At Alton Slough sometimes a score of craft do their wintering. In summer the sloughs harbor houseboats and shanty boats. These we saw also at the mouths of tributary rivers such as the St. Croix. In the abandoned canals by which boats used to go around the Upper and Lower Rapids I noted what seemed to be several derelict packets.

Over some of the sloughs and the backwaters and swamps that lead off from them there hangs a fading memory and perhaps the ghost of an odor compounded of raw whisky and cheap perfume. In their time the sloughs were part of one of the nation's frontiers. Lawless men have always flocked to the edge of things; but in a mining camp, sooner or later, there was law, even if only lynch law. It was different in the dubious backwaters of the river, for the Mississippi was itself a boundary line between states, and men—and women—whom the law would lay its hand upon needed only to cross from one bank to the other in order to escape jurisdiction.

So there came into being the floating dance hall which was also a saloon and a brothel. It might be just a pair of flatboats joined together and covered with one-story buildings, such as Charles Edward Russell saw as a boy at Davenport and which, as he recites, had "a generic name not to be repeated in print." Thieves, female harpies, and men who would do murder for a meed were aboard these floating dives. Their chosen victims were the rude raftsmen and lumbermen who at winter's end had come out of the valleys of the six great timber rivers in response to the primal urges of lust and liquor. Among the victims was an occasional town inhabitant of better social rank, of the sort that Proverbs characterizes as "a youth devoid of understanding." About the only thing to be said for the predaceous hosts and hostesses is that they used to sing "Buffalo Gals," which is a good song.

With thicker settlement, the floating resorts, also called "love boats," disappeared. They never quite came back, but there was something rather like them during prohibition, and still moonshine is made in sloughs and swampy woods behind some of the islands. Somehow stagnant water and righteous living never got along well together.

To another almost clandestine and yet innocent and worthy enterprise I gave some attention. Now and then I saw small mussel boats moving along the Mississippi's shore or coming out of one of its tributaries. They were flat-bottomed, each with a rack over it on which were hung two iron bars with a hundred or more stout crowfoot hooks suspended by short trot-lines. Mussels lie in the mud or gravel of the river's bottom with their valves slightly open; they close them tightly when a hook enters, and are brought to the surface. So in a sense this industry goes on out of sight, seems obscure, and in fact is little remarked upon. Yet it is important, because every man who has half a dozen shirts and half a dozen suits of underwear in his bureau drawers uses at least a hundred pearl buttons a year. These were once the shells of fresh-water mussels.

The fishery is called clamming, or shelling. It is almost a monopoly of the Mississippi and its affluents. Mussel shells in the rivers draining to the Atlantic can be used only for lime stucco, poultry grit, and road metal. Those in the Mississippi Valley are worked up into buttons which have the luster of pearls.

Shelling is a profitable business. A single day's catch by a sheller on Lake Pepin netted him fifty-four dollars. In one year more than fifty million pounds of shells, with a value of more than a million dollars, were taken from the Mississippi basin and transformed into buttons and novelties with a value of about eight million dollars. Along the Iowa coast for nearly two hundred miles there are button factories, with Muscatine leading, where the industry began half a century ago. I have seen mussel shells—indeed, I had one—from which as many as a dozen button blanks had been stamped.

As a veteran riverman put it to me, the shells go to the factories, the meat—which is lightly cooked in the process of detaching the shells—goes to the poultry yard and pig-pen, and any pearls are clear profit. These used to be marketed under the false name of oriental pearls but now carry their own colors. Sometimes they are found as often as one to twenty shells, sometimes as rarely as one to a hundred thousand. They are known to the trade as true pearls, baroques, slugs, and chicken feed. True fresh-water pearls are of regular form—round, oval, pear-shaped, or dewdrop—and if lustrous, translucent, and agreeably colored, command a good price. In one year, when the catch of shells in the Mississippi River and Great Lakes

region brought the fishermen a million and a quarter
dollars, the pearls and slugs taken were valued at nearly
one-tenth that sum.

Our own boat saluted every craft of consequence which
it met or overhauled, and was saluted in return. It whistled also when it approached a bridge, a lock, or a landing.
Of landings we made few, but in addition to the twenty-
six locks there were forty-eight bridges to be whistled at
going and coming. Sometimes these were approached in
the dead of night and from lonely places, the hollow hooting of our whistle echoing from shore to shore, to die
away at last in deep draws of the hills. It had two tones,
sounded together—for some reason called bells—and in
their blended salutation were notes of both comradeship
and arrogance; perhaps the word is amiable defiance.

Until a year or so ago, each river had its own code of
signals. Now every boat anywhere must give one long
blast when nearing a bridge with a lift or a draw. Sometimes it goes under a fixed span; sometimes the middle
span swings open, or rises vertically; twice there were railroad bridges with a pontoon section that was floated to
one side while we went through. At the Minnesota town
of Hastings was a bridge with a quaintly spiral approach,
cars climbing up and around a sort of tower to reach the
level that took them to the other bank.

Each boat had its own signal when blowing for a landing, this its theme song. Our own signal was one long, two
shorts, one long and one short. Approaching a lock the
Golden Eagle conformed to government orders with a long
blast followed by a short. When it met another boat the
downstream boat had right of way, sounding one blast if it
would go to the right, two if to the left.

In passing locks our boat, in a manner of speaking, was

on an ascending staircase, climbing three hundred and twenty-six feet while it traveled six hundred and fifty-six miles between St. Louis and St. Paul. Steps averaged twelve feet in height, and each was followed by perhaps twenty-five miles of level water; in winter, when ice covered the upper river, these reaches might well be called long flagstones. At Keokuk the lift was thirty-eight feet, and we entered the narrow lock chamber as into the dank gloom of the Catacombs. All locks have a uniform length of six hundred feet. Usually the gates swung backward, but at Quincy they submerged. When they came up again, unwary fish came up upon them, and these the shore blacks scrambled for.

When we neared a lock the two landing stages—in the Mississippi, boats have always had a pair of them—rose in air to the thunder of windlasses. People greeted friends on shore. Mail was handed on and off at the end of a bamboo fishing pole. At one place a yellow-haired girl baby with a cough was also handed off by her parents into the arms of the grandmother, only to be retrieved, in restored health, a day or so farther upstream. My lasting impression of the locks, however, was that a Mississippi pirate would be in bad luck nowadays, for every pool between dams was a tight prison from which he could only escape overland.

CHAPTER XVII

BETWEEN BATTLEMENTED CRAGS

NEAR the mouth of the Illinois and for some distance beyond, and again for about two hundred miles below St. Paul, the Mississippi River flows between high bluffs which challenged the gaze on our way upstream on the *Golden Eagle*. Few persons seem to know much about them. One cannot comprehend them by standing upon them and looking down at the water. He must get down and look up and keep on looking for several days while a boat takes him places. Nobody did this for nearly a generation because it could not be done.

Beltrami, Italian explorer, who went with the *Virginia* in 1823 on the first steamboat trip from St. Louis to St. Paul—this I was repeating more than a century later—was excited by what he saw. His mind, filled with Old World images, called up inevitable comparisons. The Piasa Bluff made him fancy he was viewing the palaces of Pompey and Domitian on a lake near Rome. Farther up the river he saw lofty rocks which appeared to be towers, steeples, dwellings. I shall call them battlements. The bluffs, which are from four hundred to six hundred feet high, begin with woodland below and end with woodland above. Between these green spaces the naked cliffs rise sheer in a semblance of stockades, bastions, and a regular line of fortified walls that almost subjugate the imagination into accepting them for reality. Any steamboat captain could convince a credulous tourist from overseas that these were defense works of a forgotten barbarian empire.

I shall not multiply vain words about them. The battle-mented Mississippi in some of its upper reaches has a splendor beyond speech.

The bluffs were always there, and others besides Beltrami have described them, though few as well. But the river on which they looked is almost unknown to the country. It did not resume its ancient estate until two years ago when a great series of locks and dams, completed, brought back the majesty which may have been its own in some cycle of abundant rainfall, when it flowed through unbroken forests and only the birchbark canoe of the Indian left a tremulous wake on the water.

Before this transformation was wrought, the Mississippi had been like all other American rivers, save those in whose lower courses the tides come and go. In turn each year it was prince and pauper, moving in the shortest of spans from magnificence almost to insignificance. Government reports tell the story. In Christmas week, 1871, there was just one foot of water at Cairo, where the Ohio comes in. On a day in January, 1931, there was less than four feet of water at St. Paul. On the last three days of August, this as late as 1934, there were only ten inches at Prairie du Chien. At St. Paul, head of navigation, the average volume of water in the Mississippi has been only one-tenth the maximum volume and the latter two hundred and thirty times the minimum volume. There is, or used to be, ten times as much water in the river at St. Louis as at St. Paul.

These fantastic contrasts have become ancient history. The Des Moines and Rock Island Rapids have disappeared, and with them that interesting race of men, the pilots who took boats through them. There can still be high water, but not very low water. The locks and dams take care of that. A dependable channel with a uniform depth of nine feet, usually ten or more, runs between the two big cities. Only one thing keeps the Upper Mississippi from being an all-year-round waterway, as the Ohio is. That is ice. For three months of the year, beginning with December, it is closed to navigation from St. Louis up. Farther north, from Rock Island to St. Paul, it is frozen over in severe winters for five months, beginning with November.

I saw it in summer. Broad, brimming, bank-full, it swung between haughty battlements or moved beside gently sloping shores, shadowed by oaks, beeches, maples, sycamores, willows, now and then a white-armed birch. Damming had created numerous islands, all but drowned the old wing dams with which it had been sought to control the channel, here and there marooned a house and barn that once had dry land around them. Through the low-lying woods ran long water-streets like canals. On the very edge of the river were trees which it had undermined and which were destined to topple in and become items in the ancient river litany—"snags, planters, and sawyers"— for snagboats to grapple with. Their naked roots were like fingers clutching at nothingness.

This watery wilderness, fair to the eye of man, must look good to other creatures. It is alive with fish and fowl. In the twilight I saw what may have been sunfish leaping at willow flies along the darkening shores. I heard tales of big buffalo fish, and catfish the size of small sharks. Among other finny tenants of the Mississippi are muskies, suckers, wall-eyed pike, red horse, sheepsheads, bluegills, crappies, perch, bream, small-mouthed bass, and drumfish.

Illinois and Iowa are important corn states and the wild ducks know it. I remarked a string of islands where considerable flocks in their fall migrations halt for weeks to

feed among the shocks. Farther upstream I saw smaller
flocks winging low over the water. While great blue herons
were everywhere, only now and then did I observe the
small green heron which Kentucky folk know as the fly-
up-the-creek. One wooded island which we passed toward
dusk was the haunt of black-crowned night heron, thousands of them nesting there; a few of them were flying in
and out of the trees. These birds are waders. They like
marshes and do much of their feeding at night, foraging
on crayfish, minnows, frogs, and field mice. They have
shorter necks than the blue heron, larger bodies than
the ill-named shitepoke.

I saw one flight of those clamorous creatures, the sand-
hill cranes; four crows in convocation upon a sand bar;
a procession of white cranes disappearing down a back
street of water; a great heron on its nest; tern scouting
the water; various unidentified fowl which were declared
to be jacksnipe, this seeming to be an all-inclusive term.
Once three eagles were noted circling above high crags.
Later, perhaps in the next township, another eagle crossed
the river overhead, flying from Wisconsin into Iowa. Still
later a prairie chicken crossed in the opposite direction.

Both shores have become game refuges, the government
taking title to lands flooded by its dams and establishing
sanctuaries upon them. I was told that timber wolves hide
in the hills in summer and in winter come down to the
river to dig out muskrats for tidbits.

One incidental item of wild life on the Mississippi I
have yet to record. "They are strongly attracted to light,"
concludes a printed account of a genus of small creatures
called Ephemera. Testimony to this came when we entered
the lock at Keokuk. In the rays of our searchlight I saw
what seemed to be a golden tapestry. Strange insects were

in such rapid motion that each appeared to be a maenadic procession rather than a single individual. On the southern shore of Lake Erie they are called Canadian soldiers, which is no term of compliment to a northern neighbor. Along the Mississippi they are known as willow flies. Other names are shad flies, May flies, day flies. Their adult life is only for a few hours, or at most a few days, whence the name. They are delicate creatures with membranous wings, atrophied mouth parts, and a pair of long, slender filaments at the end of the abdomen. They cannot bite, they do not eat, they do nothing at all but mate and die. The eggs, returned to the water, become larvae and pupae, and after from one to three years, during which time valuable food fishes batten upon them, the survivors come to the surface, split their skins, and fly into the night.

Does light complete the process of emergence? It would almost seem so, for on several nights every flash of the searchlight brought waves of ephemerids aboard, these appearing to rise out of the black river itself. Whenever it happened, passengers took it on the run and all lights on deck were doused. At Muscatine I heard that people were throwing them off the bridge with snow shovels, the bridge approaches so slippery that cars could not travel them. On the boat their visits were less of a nuisance than ashore and, of course, they were found only in one zone of the river. As winged embodiments of the Will to Propagate, as frenzied light-worshipers, and as literally creatures of an hour, they offered material for edifying reflection.

Viewing a beautiful, interesting, and nearly unknown river, I was reminded of a former chapter in its history. Just as in the eighteenth century there was a Grand Tour which young Englishmen of gentle blood took with their tutors along the Rhine, into Italy, and then to France, so there was a Fashionable Tour which nineteenth-century Americans took on the Mississippi. The artist George Catlin gave it a name and its itinerary. It was by steamboat to St. Louis, to the Falls of St. Anthony, back to Prairie du Chien, and thence on the Wisconsin River to Green Bay on Lake Michigan, whence a steamship took passengers past the Island of Mackinac, down Lake Huron and across Lake Erie to Buffalo and Niagara Falls. Fashionable folk from the East did take this trip from about 1835 until the Civil War. Steamboat captains used to bring Indians aboard for them to gaze at. Luxurious passenger boats were built to accommodate the traffic, and excursion parties came also from the Ohio and the lower river.

With the Mississippi again navigable and—save for the absence of pictorial Indians—more attractive than before, it may well be that with a less rococo name, the Fashionable Tour could be revived.

However, our own tour of the river involved us in a paradox. Our jack staff was set on the North Star. It might as well have been the Dog Star. The farther north we went, the hotter we found it. For the last eight of our ten days upstream and back, canicular days all of them, the temperatures reported by towns on both banks of the Mississippi were around a hundred. The heat wave was country wide, as newspapers told us. Because we were in motion and upon water, we may have been cooler than anybody else; but this is not saying we were cool. The prevailing wind was from the southwest, a following wind as we went upstream. It was a headwind on our return, and that was better.

The weather is noted because of its effect on steamboat society, society being everywhere largely a matter of clothes. All the men went about in shirt sleeves. One or two of the younger men, hairy specimens they were, stripped themselves to the waist, though they wore a little more at meals. Pictorial effects were achieved by young women, and usually on the hurricane deck. They wore shorts and swim suits and sun suits, and naïve ensembles of halters and bathing trunks, and their slacks might be called breeches of decorum, to borrow perhaps from Bill Nye. Nothing save their tresses seemed completely covered, these often with a red or blue bandana. Their other areas grew browner each day, toward the end approaching the quadroon coloring which is every summer girl's summer goal—a consummation viewed with evident satisfaction by the sepia-hued stateroom maids.

There was also steamboat society on the lower deck, where the roustabouts congregated. Their patois was unique, their patio a cleared space in the bow amid coal heaps scarcely blacker than themselves. There they loafed, gossiped, threw dice, studied the river, now and then burst into song. From the rail above we could watch them. One day a large dishpan was filled with water, flour was sifted in to make it opaque, and silver quarters, donated by passengers, were scattered on the bottom; various roustabouts, ducking their heads, brought up the coins between their teeth—not what one would call refined amusement, but an old custom on Mississippi boats. Elsewhere we saw little of these primitive, powerfully built folk except when we went ashore at night. Then we followed a devious path through the boat, in and out among coal bunkers and disused cattle pens in a gloom half lighted by the open furnace doors and by dim lanterns in the hands of the blacks.

Roustabouts have a pride of calling, a contempt for shore blacks, and among themselves a number of social ranks based on the nature of their service. At the bottom are the hillmen who carry freight on their shoulders. Above them in ascending order are the line-carriers who make the boat fast, the inside men who determine where the freight is to be stored, the freight picker who selects the items that are to go off at the next landing, and two deck hands who make these ready to put ashore. Often one of their number is a clergyman. When our vessel was in the regular packet trade, carrying freight as well as passengers, it had forty roustabouts. Larger steamboats, like the *J. M. White,* the *Robert E. Lee,* and the *Natchez,* carried about a hundred.

Of course, the steamboat's cocktail lounge, downstairs in a corner of the lowest deck, did well among a lot of us, though demand was for lemonade and beer rather than for the strong liquors of which it had a stock. It was a cubbyhole with a small bar, two chairs, two tables, two leather-covered corner benches, two electric fans. Just back of the partition were the engine, coal bunkers, and dripping paddle wheel of the packet. Yet the lounge, so small that a dozen passengers crowded it, had appeal. For one thing, it served free lunches at night—crackers and cheese and thin sausage slices—a nostalgic touch that some of us valued. It also sold chewing tobacco. On the wall was a colored Currier and Ives print, "A Midnight Race on the Mississippi," (this between the packets *Natchez* and *Eclipse*).

A curious Cape Cod weatherglass, which had place of honor back of the bar, evoked memories of the Yankee clippers of the 1850's. It was quite like a small glass kettle with a slender spout and was partly filled with red water. When the water rises slowly to the top of the spout, a general storm is approaching, but perhaps a whole day off; when it rises rapidly to the top of the spout a local storm is coming; when it bubbles out of the spout, that storm is very near; when it sinks rapidly below the top of the spout during a storm, the worst is almost over. When the water holds steady at halfway up the spout, that means clear weather.

I add a prognostication of my own: When shutters are suddenly drawn down over the array of crystal bottles and glasses of the bar, that means the boat has halted and its gangplank is in touch with shore. Then it is subject to state laws instead of federal, and where a vendor's federal license costs only twenty-five dollars on a boat in motion, state tavern laws charge hundreds of dollars for selling goods when boat and bank have so much as a plank between them.

To the hot spell I owe memorable nights on the hurricane roof. After sunset this was always comfortable and there those of us gathered who did not care to play lotto or other ship's games on the deck below, or to dance quite all the time. I call the hurricane deck the hurricane roof because Captain Buck did, and because it makes Walt Whitman's line, "I open my scuttle at night and see the far-sprinkled systems," fit exactly. Scuttle is defined as "a small opening in a vessel's deck," and also as "an opening in a roof." Either way the word met our case, though the poet was speaking only of a house roof. From the hurricane deck, with the boat darkened around and below us so the pilot could steer through the night, we saw the far-sprinkled systems, and divined other systems beyond

them. It is one of the three best places in the world for
stargazing, the two others being an upland pasture and
the seashore.

There was the full moon to make a wistful pathway
over the water; but after a night or two it was a sagging
moon which rose late, so that the stars had the show to
themselves. The procession of summer constellations across
the sky's velvety darkness was a matter to see and remember. Among them flowed the Milky Way, like the Ocean
Stream of myth-making geographers who lived a good
while ago. At intervals stars were falling, and always they
plunged into the Galaxy. Felicity, I felt, might be defined
as something to be found on the hurricane deck of a slow-
moving packet, while stars were falling through the summer night and frogs piping, crickets chanting, from shores
in shadow.

Once, just before dawn, I went out on deck to see the
winter constellations come up in the east, the Twins of
Jove leading the parade. Low in the west the moon was a
golden wedge. A chill wind was wafted from the willows.
Forward on the port side of the packet I saw the captain
nodding in an armchair, and a surge of admiration rose
within me as I realized that he had been on watch all
night long.

Not his the task of finding and following the channel;
that was the pilot's. But whenever the boat entered a lock,
its master went into hoarse-throated action, giving the
megaphoned commands that snubbed his craft against
the chamber walls and held it securely until the massive
gates swung open in front and it moved into higher water.
There were twenty-six locks, and by common report the
captain—a son of the Lower Mississippi and of open water
—hated them all equally. Yet with almost loving care he

put his charge through them, not for fear of cracking the
lock or jamming its gates, but so that no mischief might
be done the boat's wooden timbers, and none befall the
folk she carried.

So we journeyed north, while days followed nights, hills
advanced and retreated, states came and went. The river
was at least a mile broad. Its current had cleared, perhaps
because farmers had ceased plowing between their corn
rows, and there had been a dry spell. Although the entrance of streams which flowed through red clay banks—
usually these were from Wisconsin—would trouble its
waters for a spell, above them it would gleam again in
long crystal reaches that to the eye were green sometimes,
sometimes blue.

On both banks this was good farm country. Drought
had laid a withering hand on pastures, but the ranks of
Indian corn, just coming into tassel, stood high and thick.
Wheat fields, some of them with the grain already cut
and shocked, had a thrifty look; and is there more engaging color than the delicate shade of their straw and stub-
ble? Farm animals sought relief from heat in the river.
Horses and cattle stood flank deep in water. White hens
marshaled their broods beside it. Once at milking time I
saw a shepherd dog round up a herd of half-submerged
Herefords, and when they were safely headed toward the
barn, forget all about his task and take a long swim. I
thought of that dog when I saw girl swimmers, in towns
too small to afford bathhouses, modestly undressing in
the willows.

Wide as was the river, the channel swung from side to
side—crossings, they are called—bringing us so near to
shore that I caught the impudent blue of the jaybird's
coat in a stretch of woodland, heard in the fields the

cicada's song to summer, and saw bedizened butterflies idling above a painted garden. Always the scent of sweet clover was in the air.

In the evening hour the shore was a haunting thing, for then the trees, the sky, and the white, drifting clouds all were mirrored in the water, another world coming into being with no curse of reality upon it. Here I tested and affirmed the singular discovery that the designs and symmetries of the totem pole, and a number of harmonious patterns in Aztec and Oriental art, must have come from reflections of the shore in clear water as viewed at right angles to normal vision. In the gazing glass of the water I saw indubitable totem poles loom and pass.

When I turned my gaze to the shore itself, I saw there something which had no harmony of pattern yet did have a disturbing semblance of life. Along the Mississippi the surviving ranks of what once were great stands of hardwood form a screen which the eye seeks to penetrate as if to glimpse what once was behind them. When the pioneers strode westward through the aisles of sunlight and shadow, did they take with them racial memories of other forests, for ages the abode of nameless fear? Folk lore has much to say of these. The strange shapes that trees assumed, the shadows beneath them, have put a spell on the imagination of men. Once upon a time—simple words but with magic in them—all forests were enchanted. They had become a refuge for the peoples of the old mythologies. Their witches, giants, gnomes, and goblins were degenerate embodiments of Pan, the dryads, the fauns, and satyrs. Let one stand for all—the Old Man of the Woods, lame, hairy, green-eyed, itinerant, a mocker, misleader, and seducer; in him were traces of the lame Lemnian, of Wotan the Wanderer, above all of Olympian Jove.

I call up these forest shapes from their sleep in fading folk lore, because I seemed to find them along the Mississippi's shores, wherever the trees came down to the water —together with others that have no literature and no name. My quest began some years before when I was going up the Illinois. On the packet was a very old man with two tall, handsome daughters, or perhaps granddaughters, for they were not yet of middle age. The three kept to themselves and usually talked in some unknown tongue which I thought might be Indian, perhaps Choctaw, once the lingua franca of tribes and traders in the lower South. I overheard the old man say but one thing in English. He said that the trees which overhung the river were as shadowy herds of buffalo, or still larger creatures, slaking their thirst in the water.

Ever since I have watched the wooded shores of rivers— usually with half-closed eyes—when passing between them. So I did at intervals on a Mississippi voyage of more than a thousand miles. Sometimes the shapes that I saw had the semblance of dancing figures which swept along the bank without heed of the water. More often it seemed as if they were under some sorcery that held them back while urging them toward it; they were approaching the brink but not attaining it, essaying and never achieving, and endlessly moving on. Old men leaning on staffs, withered crones, girls with sportive feet, wistful priestesses of woodland dubieties—these peopled the procession. But there were other, stranger and yet recognizably human figures, stooped, crouching, with shoulders hunched, antediluvian, drawing back affrighted from their own reflections in water which still they sought. Among them also were in-human shapes—rearing snakeheads, shadowy behemoths, dragon forms, ghosts of creatures that nature undertook to fashion and put aside unfinished.

As I take it, all the forest folk of legend come out on the brink of rivers and are still to be seen there. The lore of enchanted woods, grotesque, awesome, yet richly poetic, may have had its origin in the minds of men who looked upon them from moving water a long time ago.

CHAPTER XVIII

REDSKINS

ST. PAUL was different as we divined before our boat brought us there. Near the lower end of the Mississippi, early Americans, in the woods or just out of them, found a joyous French city with plenty of things to see, and a market in which they could exchange their corn, pork, and whisky for the wares and luxuries of Europe. Besides, New Orleans was downstream, and loaded flatboats went thither for a generation before steamboats became common. At the upper end of the navigable Mississippi, when the first steamboat anchored below the Falls of St. Anthony in 1823—a century after New Orleans had become a French territorial capital —the *Virginia's* passengers found only an Indian village, an American fort, and a collection of squatters' huts which as late as 1840 was called Pig's Eye.

This was St. Paul, no outlet to Old World civilization, but just an outpost in the unpeopled wilderness; and besides, it was upstream from the settled country and flatboats go only downstream. Situated at opposite cardinal points, the two terminals shaped the growth of steamboating traditions which had cardinal points of difference. For the Upper Mississippi I find them nearly all summed up in a single pioneer word—redskins. Across the Lower Mississippi the Five Civilized Tribes passed into exile; but of the Indians upon it only the Natchez, a sun-worshiping folk whose howls brought in the day, made any history. That was more than two centuries ago. The French at-

tacked their Louisiana fort and sold the prisoners as slaves
in the West Indies, survivors taking refuge with other
tribes. There is now no Natchez nation. On the Upper
River the Indian saga is far more varied and, of course,
more recent. Abraham Lincoln—men still alive have seen
him—was a captain in the Black Hawk War.

Slowly this sense of savage backgrounds grew upon me
as the *Golden Eagle* moved northward. A multitude of
musical place- or stream-names suggested it, as well as such
rugged ones as Keokuk (Watchful Fox), friend of white
men, whom the Black Hawk party liquidated when it got
the chance. Such aboriginal appellations as Winnebago,
Menominee, Maquoketa, and Winona stand up well
enough beside pioneer names like Whisky Run, Bloody
Run, Jim Crow Island, Nigger Island, Bad Axe River,
Hanging Dog Creek, Smallpox Creek, Deadman's Slough,
and Smoot's Chute. At Rock Island I saw a statue of
Black Hawk, erected in one of those expiatory moods
to which the superior race is prone after war with another
race is ended. At Prairie du Chien, a few miles above the
mouth of the Wisconsin, we passed what had once been a
frontier fur town of consequence, with a fort, the memory
of a gay French society, and a market place where voyageurs from distant waters and Indians from the woods
trafficked in whisky, muskets, and skins.

Near the outset of the nation's contacts with the Mississippi tribes a steamboat figures. Loaded with American
troops it ended the Black Hawk War in a battle fought
in August, 1832, on the Mississippi below the mouth of
Bad Axe River. The Sacs and Foxes were trying to cross
the Mississippi in order to return to their reservation in
Iowa, after a foray in Illinois to revisit lands they still
regarded as their own. The boat got in between. Black

Hawk sent it a messenger with a flag of truce, offering to give himself up. The flag was fired upon and fighting began between the troops on the boat and the Indians on the shore. Three hundred of the latter were killed or drowned, three hundred more crossed the river during or after the fight. Thus accounts were squared for the other major incident of the war, when Black Hawk, with forty warriors, ambushed and then charged into the open upon Isaac Stillman's command of three hundred and forty volunteers, who promptly ran away. That battlefield bears the appropriate name of Stillman's Run.

Black Hawk, himself a Sac, fought on the side of the British in the War of 1812. As was the case with most Indian chiefs, he was fond of the French, respected the British but did not like them, and hated the Americans. Undoubtedly the Sacs and Foxes, in meetings where much whisky flowed, had signed treaties ceding their lands east of the Mississippi in return for an annuity, and one of these treaties Black Hawk himself signed without grasping its full purport. His case may be rested upon two sentences in his autobiography: "My reason teaches me that land cannot be sold . . . Nothing can be sold but such things as can be carried away." It was the Indian tribal code.

An industry discovered and first developed by savages gave steamboating on the Upper Mississippi a sound economic footing. This was the mining and melting of lead. As early as 1810 the Fox Indians, working under a French entrepreneur, were melting four hundred thousand pounds a year along the Fever River in Illinois, and a few years later flatboats began to take it down to St. Louis. That river changed its ill-omened name to Galena, and on it, a dozen miles from the mouth, arose the town of Galena,

Grant's home before the Civil War. It became the lead capital.

The mines in that valley and in adjacent Wisconsin and Iowa had annual yields which reached more than a million and a half dollars, or five times the value of the fur trade at St. Louis. In a single year there were one hundred and seventy-six steamboat arrivals at the Port of Galena. In the quarter century from 1823 to 1848 there were three hundred and sixty-five different steamboats on the Upper Mississippi, two hundred of them largely engaged in freighting lead. In the same period more than seven thousand steamboat trips were made to the lead mines. Now lead is taken chiefly from the Rocky Mountains where the ores have silver in them; the population of Galena has shrunk to less than four thousand and no steamboat whistle is heard on its river.

Besides Sac and Fox, other Indian peoples along the Upper Mississippi were the Sioux, Chippewas, Winnebagoes, Menominees, Iowas, and Otos. Though now and then painted warriors took a shot from the bank at a passing steamboat, they were a godsend to navigation. This was for more substantial reasons than because tourists traveled north to see skin-clad, feather-crested savages and to applaud their village dances. Because of the Indian populations, there were American forts to mount guard, soldiers to man the forts, supplies to be taken to the soldiers, annuities to the Indians, delegations of Indian chiefs to be brought to Washington to consult the Great White Father, and mass movements of savages to councils where treaties were to be signed, or to new hunting grounds farther west. All these tasks called for steamboats.

The posts where troops were stationed were Fort Madison, Fort Clarke, and Fort Atkinson in Iowa; Fort Edwards below the Lower Rapids; Fort Armstrong below the Upper Rapids; Fort Crawford at Prairie du Chien (both Zachary Taylor and Jefferson Davis were officers there); Fort Winnebago on the Wisconsin; Fort Ridgely, Fort Ripley, and Fort St. Anthony in Minnesota, the latter now Fort Snelling, at the junction of the Minnesota and Mississippi in St. Paul. From the river at Rock Island I saw Fort Armstrong, a small log blockhouse on a bluff with ancient cannon pointed over the water. In the military reservation of Fort Snelling I saw the round stone keep built in 1820.

Though there was a violent Sioux uprising during the Civil War, and eight hundred white settlers along the upper reaches of the Minnesota River lost their lives in it, none of these forts seems ever to have been attacked. Yet in time of peace steamboats sometimes had more revenue from the transport of soldiers and their supplies to the army posts than from their passenger business. The annuities to Indians, always in the form of goods brought up from St. Louis, were a major freight item. In 1844 the value of goods for the Winnebagoes alone was nearly one hundred thousand dollars.

Perhaps the most engaging chapter in the story of the steamboat concerns the dealings of government with the rude nations of the North. After their first alarms had subsided the Indians manifested a pronounced liking for the ease and comforts of steamboat travel. It was policy to keep them in friendly mood and to impress them with the power of the nation whose wards they were. What would now be called good-will trips by water were arranged for them. Sometimes large parties were taken down the Missouri and up the Mississippi to powwows called to compose tribal quarrels.

When the Winnebagoes removed to Crow Wing River in 1848, two thousand had a steamboat ride of a hundred miles north to St. Paul. It was alleged that many paddled back and for a second time were taken up the river. Some years afterward a number of their nation in Minnesota, who were to be removed to Nebraska, refused to go overland. So the government took them by "fire canoe" down the Minnesota and Mississippi and up the Missouri River —a trip nearly ten times as far. Petersen's account, based on old newspaper files, of the policy of shaping Public Relations with Savages by using steamboat techniques is good reading.

There were other chapters in upper river steamboating: the fur trade, which more than a century ago was worth a million dollars a year to St. Louis, its capital; the ferrying of westward-bound American emigrants across the Mississippi; the carrying of troops to Civil War battlefields; the movement of wheat downstream as Scandinavian farm folk made themselves new homes in the Northwest; growing excursion and tourist traffic. River trade was a vivid thing, prosperous, and acclaimed at the head of navigation. The arrival in spring of the first boat at St. Paul was eagerly awaited, publicly celebrated, rewarded by free dockage for that season.

Boats that reached there had to come up a singular lake, half a day's ride below. It took our boat the better part of three hours to navigate it. Lake Pepin is named from some unidentified Frenchman, certainly not from Pepin the Short, bastard son of Charles Martel and sire of Charlemagne. Twenty-five miles long and in places nearly four miles wide, it is larger than most of New York's Finger Lakes, far larger than Itasca, titular source of the Mississippi. Unlike many so-called lakes which have collected behind dams, it is nature's handiwork. Here and nowhere else, instead of swinging from a bluff on one shore to a bluff miles downstream on the other, the Upper River fills all the space between its barrier crags.

Long I gazed upon this lake while sitting at the evening meal on deck. So wide it seemed that almost I could have fancied myself on a bay of Huron. The shows of sunset were on the water, the far-off wooded banks were good to see. Yet the captain was wary and watched the weather, for the other name of Pepin is Lake of Tears. Flat-bottomed, light-draught steamboats with freeboards rising only a foot or so above the water were made to move on rivers where wind and wave can get no running start, and in heavy gales boats can make for the willows, seldom more than a pair of furlongs distant. Sometimes in rough weather, lake waves are a dozen feet high—and there are no natural harbors where boats can put in. To meet that lack the government has built two wind havens where they can seek refuge. Not always have they found it or ridden out the storms. Half a century ago the excursion steamer *Sea Wing* capsized with two hundred passengers aboard, and ninety-seven of them were drowned. In another storm a packet lost its chimneys. In another, a side-wheeler was thrown clear on its beam-ends, one of the wheels revolving in air; but somehow it righted itself. Still other and minor and seemingly unrecorded wrecks have given the basin the name of a graveyard.

In days when steamboating was at its height Lake Pepin retarded the opening of spring navigation.[1] When the ice broke along the Lower River reaches every packet loaded up with passengers and freight and headed for St. Paul. In the lake, ice held for a week or fortnight longer than in the

[1] Petersen's *Steamboating on the Upper Mississippi*, p. 451 *et seq.*

river at either end of it. Sometimes as many as a score of packets, with thousands of persons aboard, lay at the foot of Pepin, waiting for the ice to go out. There are tales of passengers helping to chop a channel through it, of other passengers who walked ashore over the ice and on to Red Wing, where packets from the Minnesota River carried them to St. Paul ahead of the boats on which they had first taken passage.

In 1854 the first railroad reached the Mississippi. By 1860 seven of its ports had rail connections with the Atlantic seaboard. By 1867 St. Paul itself was thus linked with the Great Lakes. Until the seventies all this helped steamboating, for there was no north-and-south railroad line between St. Louis and St. Paul, and immigrants brought to river ports had to complete their journey by boat. By 1890, however, the Mississippi packets generally had succumbed to railroad competition for the freight and passenger trade.

Another river institution began to dwindle at about the same time. I had rather expected to find rafts on the Upper Mississippi, which for seventy years before and for nearly seven hundred miles had presented a panorama of floating logs. I saw none, nor along the Great River did I see any signs of the prostrated forests of which I had read. Hardwoods and not pines frame it, the second growth looking about as well as virgin timber. Until near the end of those seventy years nothing but white pine logs came down the Mississippi, and the big woods where they grew were back upon tributary rivers.

White pine had the call everywhere from the very beginning of American settlement. Pioneers made their log huts out of whatever trees were near at hand, yet chose white pine when they could get it. When sawmills came in, these worked up nothing else. The pines had straight trunks; their soft wood yielded readily to the axe, and was

easily sawed into planks and boards. When the forests of
Minnesota, Michigan, and Wisconsin were felled, their
maple and birch trees were left standing. Later, lumbermen turned to the yellow pine and cypress of the South
—and to hardwoods everywhere for vehicles, implements,
doors, pianos, furniture. But as long as the white pine trees
of the Northern forests lasted, it was their dedicated service
to make homes for the children of men.

Lumbering began in the Upper Mississippi region in
1824,[1] reached a peak in 1892, and declined rapidly thereafter, the last raft of consequence coming down the river
in 1915. The white pine woods were on the Mississippi far
above the Falls of St. Anthony; on the Wisconsin, Black,
and Chippewa, all Wisconsin rivers; on the Minnesota in
Minnesota, and on the St. Croix which is both a Wisconsin
and a Minnesota waterway. Down them in spring the logs
floated. They were cut in winter by men who lived crudely
but comfortably in large camps. The camps took pride in
the quantities of wholesome food which they set on their
tables, in the skill of their cooks, particularly in the ritual
of the bean-pot.

These camps touched the world of letters at one point,
enriching with their own hilarities the forest saga of Paul
Bunyan, wonder-working foreman first talked about in the
bunkhouses of New England and Canada; the amiable
giant who moved in a world of strange creatures like the
tote-road shagamaw, the splinter cat, and the gumberoo
which explodes when too near a campfire. Of the man himself there are so many guesses—one that his name is a corruption of Paul Bonhomme, a French Canadian—that I
venture another. Before the legend was current in print,
I read in some old book the tale of a grotesque Algonquian
god, who wrought marvels and had a name resembling

[1] Cf. Russell's *A-Rafting on the Mississip.*

Paul Bunyan's. If my surmise be correct Paul is just another Olympian.

By creeks and tote-roads and skidways, logs reached the timber rivers and were swept down their swollen current. Some went to sawmills that sprang up in all the towns on the Upper Mississippi. Others went to anchored booms where they were made up into rafts that might be a quarter of a mile long and a hundred yards wide, while drawing but a foot and a half of water. These were destined for mills in the big towns farther down. Crews of a score or more of lumberjacks, housed in rude shanties upon the rafts, manned the sweeps that kept them in their course. The capricious, island-fretted reaches of the river challenged the skill of pilots whose task it was to see that their wooden flotillas did not run aground in the chutes, or succumb to wild water in the Upper and Lower Rapids, or jam up and go to pieces on towheads.

The pilots were highly paid and proud of their calling —this proclaimed by uniforms in which slouch hats, red shirts with black silk cravats, and sometimes black gloves, were featured. As for their crews, a saying which I had heard on the Cumberland—that the beard of a raftsman would turn a razor's edge—tells nearly all that needs to be told. It has been said that the whisky they drank would take the hair from a buffalo hide. Disturbers of the peace of towns where they stopped, terrorizers of the steamboats on which they took return passage, unruly, reckless, violent, and yet useful servants of the time, their story repeated the earlier saga of flatboatmen on the Lower River.

If their wild ways need the palliatory word, and if the tale of the pineries of three states, ravaged without thought of the morrow, calls for exculpation, both are to be sought and in a measure to be found on the prairies and treeless plains beyond the Mississippi. Gone are the sod houses, those singular mimicries of log cabin models farther east. In their place are sightly and substantial frame dwellings, millions of them, with their attendant barns, and wagon sheds, and corn cribs, and trellises for summer flowers—legacies all of the Northern woods.

CHAPTER XIX

THEY BEAR TRIBUTE

BOAT stores have the tang of yesterdays, an atmosphere of sagacious leisure, a nondescript assortment of commodities. Each is at once a rendezvous for river folk and a museum of waterside history. Men who run them must do so more for love of their calling than for profits. Such establishments are becoming scarce. I saw one at the Illinois town of Quincy when our packet lay there for an hour on its trip to St. Paul. It was near the river, back of a good paved landing at the foot of a steep street which led up into the town; near-by in an island chute were numerous craft.

This was Quincy's oldest store. It was built of logs in 1822 as a trading post. The logs are still there, but under plaster. On the inner walls was the proprietor's collection of old steamboat pictures. On floors and counters were anchors, oars, fishing rods and reels, chains, lead lines, ropes and cordage, oakum, calking chisels and mallets, stocks of steamboat groceries. A boat store is a country store of about 1885 gone river-minded.

On the Iowa side and farther up, at another stop of the *Golden Eagle,* I dropped into an old river hotel near the water front of Davenport. A long, neat, three-story edifice with an office that ran its entire length, it breathed a welcome for whoever follows the Mississippi. The proprietor remembered days when steamboat captains were his patrons. He said that his wife had been a passenger on the last trip of the last Diamond Jo boat from St. Paul to St. Louis, and that, he thought, might be thirty-eight years ago. A party

of New Yorkers had come on for the occasion. I sat there
for a while to get on terms with this venerable and re-
spectable hostelry. It had good wooden chairs and writing
desks, a coffee room, a barber shop, a swinging door with
the sign "Gents" upon it, hanging maps of the United
States and of Iowa, and elsewhere on the cream-tinted walls
a large and ancient steel engraving in a gilt frame with the
legend, "Washington and His Generals." There must have
been forty of them, and all in full-dress uniform.

I pondered these generals, and then raised the case of
captains, of whom the river remembers a good deal more.
"In the old days," said a man who knew, "a steamboat captain had a public standing and a prestige hard to realize
now or to define."

"Like a mayor," I suggested.

"Better than that."

"Like a general?"

"Different from that."

"Well, what then?"

"More like a bishop, but with some difference in vocab-
ulary!"

Except in one or two instances the chief towns of the
states, along the borders of which we traveled, were on the
river. Usually a smaller river came in beside them, though
small, it might be, only in comparison with the Father of
Waters. The Missouri, Illinois, Des Moines, Wisconsin,
and Minnesota are all longer than the Hudson, but far
from as wide or deep. Whatever their size, tributary streams
have always engrossed me more than the towns that guarded
their mouths. In the long view, the confluences of rivers
have significances surpassing what men build beside them.

The backward view of those that enter the Mississippi
opens vistas in American history. Where they came in, the
frontier forts were located. So were trading posts; among

others, at the mouths of the Iowa, Des Moines, Skunk,
Fever, Wisconsin, Chippewa, and Minnesota Rivers; sometimes also, as at the Falls of the St. Croix, they were located
where a river fell far and canoes had to follow a portage
path to reach calm water above or below. Down these tributary streams came the stuffs of the forest and plains—pelts
of beaver, bear, deer, and buffalo. Every trading post was
the scene of wild and motley gatherings between red hunters and white trappers. Yet, though liquor flowed, there
were few bloody brawls, for the heads of posts were often
connected by marriage—or what passed for it—with the Indian chiefs. A social institution which in the Southeastern
states had given the tribes for leaders half-breed Scotchmen
like Osceola and John Ross, and which still flourishes at
the wilderness camps of the great Canadian fur companies,
made for peace at the trading posts of the Northwest. Besides, the truce that is over all market places was upon
them.

Most appealing to me of tributaries above the Missouri
was the Wisconsin, in some part because the trading post
of Prairie du Chien at its mouth has had the most colorful
history; in greater part because along the river ran an old
highway of trade between the Great Lakes and the Mississippi. Indian canoes came across Lake Michigan to the
head of Green Bay, went up the Fox River, and were carried over a portage to the upper Wisconsin, where they
took water again for a trip that ended at St. Louis; thence
bateaux bore their burden of pelts to New Orleans. Keelboats filled with American soldiers took the same route to
the Mississippi later on an exploring expedition. For a
while furs from the Upper Mississippi went east upon it:
but the keelboats suffered such damage from snags and
sand bars and over the rough ways of the portage that they
made St. Louis their sole destination.

Once there were steamboats on the Wisconsin. A standard atlas says that it is "navigable to Portage (a distance of two hundred miles), where a canal prolongs navigation to the waters of the northern Fox River." So once was the case, but the latest report of the Army Chief of Engineers makes no note of commercial navigation upon it.

There is, however, commercial navigation on the Rock River, another water route between the Great Lakes and the Father of Waters. This river feeds the Hennepin Canal, and on its lower reaches becomes part of it. The canal leaves the Illinois at Great Bend and enters the Mississippi at Rock Island. There are thirty-two small locks upon it, the channel at low water is six feet deep, and through it, between the Mississippi and Chicago, towboats and barges pass—in 1938 five steamers and two hundred and thirty-four barges. Some seventy miles long, it is the only considerable canal that has been built in the country since railways reached the Mississippi. When the first steamboat went up Rock River in 1836, every place which it passed gave the captain a town lot. A few years before that time the largest village of the Sacs was near the river's mouth.

The St. Croix, which for a hundred miles forms the boundary between Wisconsin and Minnesota, also has commercial navigation. Steamboats were on it early, and after a lapse of nearly a decade returned to it in 1929. There is a nine-foot channel from its mouth to the Falls or Dalles fifty miles above; upon it in 1938 there was a tonnage valued at nearly six hundred thousand dollars, the cargoes including vehicles, cattle, hogs, horses, sheep, and logs. Half a century ago it was one of the six great timber rivers.

Though De Tocqueville said that the Mississippi had

fifty-seven large, navigable tributaries, I have named here
the only two above the Missouri and Illinois that steamboats can enter. There was once a number of others. On
high water hundreds of Sioux were brought down the
Minnesota to Fort Snelling after the 1862 uprising; now
there are only two feet of mean low water in the channel
and there has been no commerce since 1920. There is one
lock but no boatable water on the Galena, once thronged
with packets. Steamboats used to go up the Des Moines
(River of the Monks) as far as Iowa's capital; they could
not now if they would. They can no longer go up the
Chippewa.

Nor can they go up or down the Red River of the
North, though, according to the books, it is navigable
from Grand Forks in North Dakota to its mouth in
Canada. I had always wondered, but had never taken the
trouble to find out, why the government pilot regulations
—as framed certificates in the cabins of various boats ap-
prised me—should group the Mississippi and its tributaries
with the Red River of the North. The Mississippi formed
part of the eastern boundary of Minnesota while the Red
River formed most of Minnesota's western boundary, and
they followed parallel courses in opposite directions hundreds of miles apart. One discharged its waters into the
Gulf of Mexico, the other eventually into Hudson Bay
by way of Lake Winnipeg.

I learned on this cruise that they are connected by way
of Lake Traverse and the Minnesota River. At high water
it is asserted that small boats can still pass from the Red
to the Upper Mississippi. Before there were steamboats
on the latter, mackinaw boats laden with provisions made
trips from Prairie du Chien, up the Mississippi to the
Minnesota, up the Minnesota to its source, and thence—
though by portage—to waters entering Red River and on

into Canada to the new Scotch settlement at Winnipeg. Supplies, however, were usually sent in oxcarts from the head of navigation on the Minnesota to the head of navigation on Red River at Grand Forks, and thence by small steamboats to their destination. The long processions of Red River oxcarts made a great name in history. With their creaking cartwheels they also made a great noise upon the prairie.

Smaller rivers were navigable at flood, as indeed were many creeks, for some of the early steamboats drew less than two feet. These streams have their own stories of canoe and flatboat traffic and still other claims to attention. There are waterfalls and picturesque gorges upon nearly all of them. Below the mouth of Bad Axe River the Black Hawk War was ended in battle. Near the mouth of the Iowa, white men—Marquette and Joliet in 1673—first saw red men on the Upper Mississippi, and there annuities for Sacs and Foxes used to be delivered. At the mouth of the Yellow River in Wisconsin stood Painted Rock, which Indians held in awe and each year adorned with a fresh coat of red and yellow. Two other small rivers, both in Iowa, have names to be noted: Wapsipinicon, which contrives to be at once ludicrous and melodious, and Skunk, perhaps the only case among river names where the French term—*Bête Puante*—sounds no better than the English equivalent.

For rivers which are called navigable but which are not, the explanation is that few, except those on which the tides range, remain navigable of their own accord. Bars form, trees fall in, boats snag and sink, bridges are built which no steamboat can get under. Falling trees call for a never-ending campaign. The records of the Army Engineer Corps tell the story. On the Mississippi I note that in one year, near the beginning of the century, "about

thirty-four thousand snags, etc., were removed." Other
items tell of pulling trees back by the hundreds, of felling
leaning trees by the thousands, of clearing away wrecks
and stumps and logs. This flotsam and jetsam the snagboats used to cut into firewood lengths so that it should
trouble no more and pile on the banks for neighboring
farmers to carry off. By such campaigns the army engineers
can make any stream navigable, but this they do only
when it is worth while.

Let alone, rivers return to a canoe past. What it means
to arrest the trend on a large river is set forth in a striking
passage in *The Oregon Trail,* in which Parkman records
his descent (1846) of the Missouri, which he had ascended
in high water: "It was fallen very low, and all the secrets
of its treacherous shallows were exposed to view. It was
frightful to see the dead and broken trees, thick-set as a
military abatis, firmly imbedded in the sand, and all pointing downstream, ready to impale any unhappy steamboat
that at high water should pass over that dangerous
ground."

In the Sioux tongue the Minnesota River, which I
glimpsed at journey's end, is "sky-tinted water." So was
the Mississippi as we swept through the sunset hour of the
last day upbound. I had seen the same spectacle on the
Dakota prairies and on the Great Lakes. Mark Twain
called the region Sunset Land. Day dies haughtily and yet
tenderly and very slowly, and after its rich colors have
faded out of the sky they deepen in the river and for a
while hold dominion there. We who were pilgrims upon
it could tilt the golden bowl of sunset and find it good
to the last drop.

Then the curtain of darkness fell. Through the hot
night we moved between glimmering shores to our dock
in St. Paul. We had started on a Tuesday afternoon. We

were in at nine o'clock Saturday night. Nor was our coming unregarded. A large moonlight excursion boat, all lights and flags, was about to start from the same small landing. It whistled, it played lively tunes on a steam calliope, it moved a bit to let us edge in. Thousands of St. Paul's inhabitants, going aboard it, cast curious glances at our small pedestrian packet.

Our sojourn at St. Paul, where we spent two nights and most of two days, is a quaint chapter in retrospect. We were almost under a big stone bridge. We were almost up against a big passenger station and a freight station. Night and day on two levels smart locomotives went clanging and boxcars went lumbering by. Along the other shore were barges, houseboats, shanty boats; also a huge and derelict menagerie boat which a year before had exhibited stuffed animals as well as live ones. Above the water flitted tern with blue bodies and sharp bills, questing for food, squealing and fighting among themselves over the choicer morsels. The temperature ashore the second day was one hundred and three in the shade.

Hour after hour people sat on the dock and watched the boat, their interest heightened when we took our meals on deck in full view of the citizenry. When bedtime came our people walked across the hurricane roof to the showers, and emerging, sat in little family groups, clad only in bathrobes and pajamas, while they cooled off, still a close-up for interested bystanders. I repeat, it was quaint. I slept soundly amid all the tumult of homing railroad trains, yet did not protest when the packet started back.

In June 1941, the *Golden Eagle* struck a hidden dike below St. Louis and sank in twelve feet of water. Prompt measures were taken to raise it.

CHAPTER XX

DOWN THE MISSOURI

THIS was another river, one which followed strange, wild laws of its own and it was about a year after I had been on the Upper Mississippi. The hour was bedtime, the place where three states meet. Crossing a bridge, the four of us shifted from Iowa into Nebraska. As we carried our bags downward through a dark woodland, South Dakota was just behind us. Below, dimly outlined by its own lamps, lay a boat of some size. Out of it a man came with a flashlight to illumine the broken path. We followed him aboard. Soon I was in a berth in a little stateroom and fast asleep. When I awoke in the small hours and went to the window I could hear a nighthawk crying overhead and the slumbrous song of frogs along the bank, and see across a swiftly moving river the lights of a sleeping city.

At daybreak the thunder of engines and the shaking of the boat's timbers aroused me. We were under way. While I was dressing for breakfast there was a sudden jar. We were aground on a sand bank, but only for a moment. The boat backed off and went on. Soon I heard a curious chanting from the deck below. It was like the bleating of lambs in a meadow, yet the voice was human. I could not get the figures it was repeating, but two phrases I caught. One was Mark Twain, which meant twelve feet of water in the channel. The other was No Bottom, which meant anything more than twelve feet. It might mean thirty or forty, for even in low water there are such depths in the river.

Had I not known where I was, had I been a prisoner instead of a guest of the army officers who brought me aboard, that bump on a bar—and there were more like it on the first day—together with the cries of the leadsman in the bow of the boat would have told me. I was on the Missouri. I had begun a six-day trip from Sioux City in the northwestern corner of Iowa to St. Louis on the Mississippi, sixteen miles below the Missouri's mouth. A journey of nearly seven hundred and eighty miles lay ahead.

Most of the route was to the south, while the Missouri performed those boundary tasks which all great rivers accept as their own, and drew parts of the state lines of South Dakota, Iowa, Nebraska, Kansas, and Missouri. But my course—and the river's—was to change lower down. I borrow from Thomas H. Benton, old-time master of the sounding phrase, the words for it: "Here, where these rocky bluffs meet and turn aside the sweeping current of this mighty river, here the Missouri, after pursuing her southern course for nearly two thousand miles, turns eastward to meet the Mississippi." He was speaking of Kansas City, and the words are on his monument there. I add that for once he did less than justice to that West which he was so wont to glorify. Counting the mountain-born, eastward-flowing Montana stretch—to which he assigned an inadequate mileage—the Missouri travels twenty-nine hundred and fifty miles, which makes it the longest of American waterways.

I come back to my first breakfast. Eight persons sat down at the messroom table in the stern of the boat, and a white-clad, white-capped steward served us with fruit juice, a cereal, eggs, toast, and coffee. Two table items intrigued me: the glass salt cellars were shaped like lighthouses, and there were narrow silver napkin bands each with a number; mine was number five. This device saves laundry bills, and why has it become so nearly disused? Of the seven other men at the table, four were civilian employees of the Missouri River Division of the War Department. The three others were the engineer officers with whom I had come aboard the night before.

Breakfast was dispatched and we were all in the pilothouse by seven o'clock in the morning, about two hours ahead of usual office hours elsewhere. It did not take long to discover that this was an inspection tour and no junket. The pilothouse was a workshop in which men who knew every mile of the river were watching it two ways— by using their eyes on water and shore, and by studying maps of both drawn on a scale of about one mile to every two inches. Those maps embodied history, current affairs, reasonable expectations, all set forth in different colors. Was a new bar forming on one of the crossings? What did that boil mean? Was the river making land behind those dikes as commanded to do, or pushing too far into a bend, or stealthily edging over to a course it had abandoned generations before, or making feints and passes toward shores it should let alone? How was work proceeding with the squads of men that were dredging and blasting and pile driving, and cutting willows to weave into mattresses?

These were no perfunctory matters. Such trips are made twice a month, and area engineers in smaller boats are on the river every day. The Missouri follows sudden impulses, beneficent or maleficent, and literally executes them overnight. It is a good-Lord, good-Devil river, and never either of them two days in succession. Wherefore, while I looked on, the men in the pilothouse held their conferences as to what it would do next and how to hinder or help it. Engineering is a game of outguessing it, but always of seeming to play along with it. Once all of it was

—as everything above Sioux City still is—what is called a wild river. On the Ohio, which is civilized, engineering is a science, on the Missouri an art presupposing some understanding of the secret minds of river gods.

When my hosts pointed out things on their maps I reminded them that while they were interested solely in the channel, my interest took in the entire river, which included also the boat we were on, the ranks of cotton-woods back of the willows along the banks, the brown hawks hunting for meadow mice, and the joy-riding grackles which swept down stream, black against the bone-white of skeleton tree trunks adrift on the swift waters. These things one could see for one's self; but I was also curious about the river's history, and there the army officers and the pilots could help, pointing out bends where packets had gone to pot, telling the story behind odd place-names.

We were on the survey boat, *Sergeant Pryor,* and going along at from eleven to thirteen miles an hour. It is one of four such boats, all named after sergeants on the Lewis and Clark Expedition. The others are the *Sergeant Floyd,* the *Patrick Gass,* and the *John Ordway.* Our craft, a Diesel boat with twin-screw propellers, was only eighty feet long by twenty-two wide. It had a net tonnage of a hundred and nine and drew four feet of water. There were towing knees in front. In the bow where the leadsman stood were coils of rope, a capstan, an anchor, and the sounding pole—a stick with alternate bars of red, white, black, and green, each a foot long. A crew of fourteen had its quarters on the lower deck. The deck above boasted of only one shower bath, but had eight comfortable bunks. Outstanding feature of our craft was its height. The pilot-house was almost a turret, its elevation giving the officers a commanding view of a river in constant need of watching. It had an old-fashioned steering wheel with spokes, but was guided by levers. On the jack staff in the bow of the boat flew a red flag with a white castle upon it, emblem of the Engineer Department. In the stern was the American flag. Both came down at sunset.

Once well under way my thoughts went back to the wild river which is beyond Sioux City, following it upward to its beginnings in western Montana more than seven thousand feet above the sea. I never had been on it, but on two counts I knew a little something about it. For days I had traveled beside it on a railroad train, and noted the way its slender channel wound beside scanty tree-borders; noted also, for I was keenly interested in cabins, the smallness of the logs—mere poles—which were built into the abodes of squaw men and squatters. Now and then I saw Indians riding along the valley paths on small, tough horses. At Great Falls in Montana the Missouri bade me a sonorous farewell and by other streams and passes I went on to the Coast.

The second count is that I had read a report of the Missouri cruise of the *John Ordway* the summer before in the *Waterways Journal* of St. Louis, whose editor, Captain Wright, was a passenger. Towing four wooden barges, it started at Fort Peck in Montana, three hundred and twenty-seven miles below Fort Benton, the historic head of navigation, and in thirteen days traveled nearly five hundred miles to Lucky Mountain, just short of Bismarck, North Dakota's capital. That was at the rate of thirty-eight miles a day.

Quaintest, perhaps, of all American travel narratives of the generation is Captain Wright's account of this journey. One would not quite say of him, as was said of Columbus, that when he started he did not know where he was going, when he reached his destination he did not know where he was, and when he returned he did not know where he had been. Yet his voyage had almost the quality of mystery of one of those voyages in quest of enchanted islands that Irish sailors made in the age of fable. While the men aboard the *John Ordway* knew where they wanted to go, they seldom knew anything else. They had no river maps, no bridge maps, and road maps shed small light on the Missouri and the settlements along it. They were always guessing the names of these settlements, mistaking other towns for Wolf Point, for example, which for some reason they were keen to see. In the Wright narrative, which runs through fifteen issues of his magazine, there are constant references to an "east-west mountain" the trend of which they followed. Apparently none of the adventurers ever learned its name.

Their course was from sand bar to sand bar. The towboat, which drew three and a half feet, was constantly running aground or into a bank, and pulling away again. It did not travel by night, which was wise. On the first day it made nineteen miles, on the second about forty-nine, and on most of the other days its mileage was somewhere between these two figures. Sample statements and phrases, taken from the record, may give the savor of this river saga: "The *Ordway* made a crossing with much rubbing and some jerking." The first whirlpool proved to be "a first-class merry-go-round." "Except for a thinning line of river-bank cottonwoods, hardly a tree had we seen in all of eastern Montana." "Whatever this 7 P.M. town might be named, it boasted a good many Indians." "The river turned south. In the distance it ran square up against the usual east-west mountain range." "Twistings, grindings, and innumerable rubbings on the bottom." "Abreast a cheerless looking town, boasting three red-colored wheat elevators. Oh, well, the name of a village is unimportant."

That mysterious mountain moves in and out of the story, "faithfully following us on the right or south river bank." "The farthest we have so far been south of Canada is less than eighty miles." "We are flanking a street-corner turn where the river fetches up against a mountain. On its summit are nine people, the largest group gathered to watch us within the past three days." There is one romantic note: "Three squaws were attired in vivid red shawls, and one of them took hers off and waved!"

Up the river down which the *Ordway* groped, and on which I was now traveling, three keelboats set forth in May, 1804. Their starting point was St. Louis, which was my destination. The Lewis and Clark Expedition was sent out by the hundred-minded Jefferson to explore the Louisiana Territory, just purchased from France, and to follow up the Missouri to its source. Before the river froze, the party had gone sixteen hundred miles. It wintered for five months near Bismarck, and when the ice ran out the thirty-two men went on, in fifty days gaining their first sight of the Rockies. They discovered the three forks of the Missouri, and named them after Jefferson, Madison, and Gallatin. In November, 1805, they reached the Pacific at the mouth of the Columbia, having gone forty-one hundred miles. The return trip brought their mileage to eighty-five hundred. Of all explorations of the American continent this was the greatest and most fruitful.

From it stems the story of the Missouri River region. The capital of the upper Missouri, and the central point in its history, was Fort Union, near the boundary of Montana and North Dakota, where the Yellowstone comes in from the South. Here in 1828 the American Fur Company set up a trading post—one of half a dozen on the upper river—with a cottonwood stockade, stone bastions for cannon, warehouses, huts for the men, and a reception room for visiting braves and their squaws.

Kenneth McKenzie was the *bourgeois,* ruling with something of the state and authority of a Highland chieftain. Among the tribes whom he is supposed to have influenced were the ever-friendly Crows, the savage Sioux, the stone-boiling Assiniboines, the Mandans of the pheasant country, the Minnetarees or Willow People, the Grosventres, who ate their buffalo sausages raw, the well-named Flatheads and Nez Percés, and the numerous and powerful Blackfeet. They came to Fort Union to trade. Noted white men came there to see or serve: the artist Catlin, the scout Jim Bridger, Prince Maximilian of Wied, De Smet the Belgian missionary. For a generation the post flourished.

Furs came to it and to other posts by water in craft of all sorts—in cottonwood pirogues, in tublike skin boats paddled by squaws, in bullboats of buffalo skins on a framework of willow poles, in keelboats, and in mackinaw boats. Steamboats appeared on the river, the *Western Engineer* getting as far as Council Bluffs in 1819. The *Yellowstone* went farther, reaching Fort Union in 1831. Thus began the most daring of all chapters in American river navigation. Risks were high, but so were profits. A single trip might bring in enough money to pay for the boat. It must needs pay for itself in three or four years, for by that time, as a usual thing, the boat was no more. Three hundred Missouri River steamboats blew up or went to the bottom. It is asserted that the wreck of one lies in every bend of the river. An army engineer told me he had seen the dredges bring up fragments of these forgotten packets, and had examined the metal of their boilers and other parts—crude and coarse-grained as if forged in some blacksmith shop in the backwoods, and so not foreordained to a long life.

For the first seventy-five years of the nineteenth century the Missouri wrote most of the history of the Northwest. Up and down it passed the pioneers and pelts of the fur trade, the garrisons of the numerous army posts strung along from Fort Randolph to Fort Benton, supplies for the troops when an Indian war was on, annuities for the Indians when they were at peace, delegations of savage orators to the treaty grounds. Also there were big-game hunters from Europe, government agents, scouts, individual trappers, gold seekers, and emigrants. The Indians always liked the traders. Steamboat men, to judge from their possibly biased narratives, thought poorly of the first swarm of emigrants, as men of little means who might not keep their covenants.

Before a railroad reached the Missouri at Jefferson City in 1855, St. Louis was the starting point of its navigation. In turn, Sioux City, Yankton, and then Bismarck superseded it. The mountain boats were nearly all low-water side-wheelers. One of them, the *Chippewa,* which ascended the tributary of Yellowstone for nearly five hundred miles, drew only twelve inches when traveling light. There were —and there are—two seasons of high water: the April rise, due to spring rains and melting snow in the lower valley; and the June rise, caused by the breaking of winter in the high Rockies. After availing of both seasons, the Missouri's steamboats left "that rainwater creek above Bismarck" (Horace Bixby's injurious phrase) when cold weather came, and shifted to the Lower Mississippi for winter service there.

Steamboats had their pilothouses and cabin decks sheathed with boiler iron against Indian bullets. When they came upon a herd of buffalo crossing the Missouri they lay by, lest one of the great brutes get entangled in a wheel. Save when there was a bright moon and some urgency was at hand they traveled only by day. In the higher latitudes their day started at three A.M. and ended at nine P.M. They burned on an average twenty-five cords of hardwood, or thirty cords of cottonwood, in twenty-four hours of steaming. On the lower river there were woodyards. On the upper river, boats depended on piles of driftwood and on standing timber which had been previously deadened. Wood sometimes sold as high as eight dollars a cord above Fort Randall. The Indians who vended it practiced tricks, sitting down in shallow water before their woodpiles to make an approaching boat believe they were standing in depths providing easy anchorage; smearing the ends of cottonwood logs with vermilion so that at a distance they could be mistaken for red cedar, which burned readily even in sap. Another source of steamboat firewood was the stockades and buildings of abandoned army posts and trading posts—which for the most part had been poorly constructed, were flooded in high water, and were overrun with rats.

Crew and passengers on an average boat numbered from one hundred to two hundred persons. The standard table fare at first was straitened—pork, hominy, navy beans. But hunters went ahead at night to kill game and hang it conspicuously along the banks. A young buffalo cow was a windfall. Passengers shot at geese and ducks while walking across the banks to meet the vessel at the next turn—a hazardous thing in Indian territory. Arrival at a trading post was a great event. So at times was the start back to St. Louis, voyageurs celebrating with a wild debauch.

Some of the cargoes were of great value, some of the profits enormous. All boats carried gold dust down. The

Luella brought two hundred and thirty miners and gold dust worth a million and a quarter dollars back to civilization. In 1866 the profits of three single voyages were $17,000, $40,000, and $65,000. This was because travel fares and freight rates were high—three hundred dollars for cabin passengers from St. Louis to Fort Benton, twelve cents a pound for freight. Pilots were paid as much as twelve hundred dollars a month. Passengers, particularly the miners and fur traders, always returned by boat, lest they be robbed and slain by Indians, cattle rustlers, or outlaws on the routes overland.

So steamboating on the upper Missouri waxed and then waned. Its golden period was between 1855 and 1860. Fast, elegant craft were put on the river, and racing was common. There were fifty-nine boats on the lower river in 1858, three hundred and six steamboat arrivals at Leavenworth. In 1860 the *Chippewa* reached Fort Benton. In 1866 the *Peter Balen* ascended thirty-one miles beyond, or to within six miles of Great Falls, farthest point ever reached under steam on the river. In the same year seven packets lay at one time at the Fort Benton levee.

The duel between the steamboats and the railroads ran from 1859 to 1887, when the Great Northern Railroad reached Helena, Montana. That was about the end. As one steamboat captain has alleged, packets began to sink with amazing regularity, 70 per cent of them from snags, and the marine insurance companies took a beating. The last commercial steamboat reached Fort Benton in 1890.

Now, with the upper Missouri and its dime-novel story of adventure and vicissitude behind me, I was going down the lower Missouri and watching the nation's effort to make it again a populous, and—for the first time—a dependable waterway.

CHAPTER XXI

CAJOLING CALIBAN

BEFORE I embarked on the Missouri I knew that it was very long and that it was whimsical; and that was about all I knew. It was small where I had seen it in Montana; full of sand bars when I saw it at Council Bluffs two years ago just before the April rise. It was also the Big Muddy of popular nomenclature. That it was a great and in places a very beautiful river—comparable to the Ohio itself—nobody had told me. On another count I may liken it to the Ohio. Before there were roads or railways each was a slanting route into an unknown continent, one into the Old West, the other into the New. On them, and on the short span of the Mississippi between them, trappers and settlers, and then an active commerce, had passed from the Appalachians clear to the Rockies.

The Missouri has been fantastically misrepresented. Of course it bears plenty of silt, as does the fructifying Nile; and at sunset its waters have the same golden hue. But this is not held against Egypt's ancient river, nor might it ever have been held against the Missouri but for somebody's ignorant excursion into etymology. No, the name is not Indian for a large and muddy river. It seems to come from the Oumessourit Indians who dwelt far down the river and to whom other tribes gave a name which meant "Living at the Mouth of the Waters." It is simply a significant place-name, like the Indian names Quapaw and Omaha which—as elsewhere noted—mean the Down-River People and the Up-River People.

For the most part I was studying the shouldering bluffs and the wild marshlands that countered them on the other side of the river, and pondering the seeming loneliness of much of the great valley. These, however, were scenic matters and of the background. In the foreground, on the river's very edge, were a number of things which seemed as whimsical as the river itself. The shores looked somewhat like inundated stockyards, somewhat like fenced cattle ranges, somewhat like roofless piers reaching out over salt water to dancing pavilions that a high tide had carried away. So-called dikes created these effects.

The dikes were not earth embankments, at least at the start. They were long rows of piles, assembled like corn in a hill in clumps of threes, and driven down twenty to thirty feet deep into the earth. Some paralleled the shore, and their purpose was to build up land behind it. Others were spurs at acute angles, their purpose to push back the shores on the other side of the river. Still others were like log pigpens with four sides, and here, because of rock bottom, the piles were horizontal instead of vertical. The piles were principally cypress trees from the bayous of the South, firs from the far Northwest. Under water they may last for thousands of years. Above it, the average life is little in excess of ten years.

The Missouri is a mason which carries along its own mortar and building materials; it is also a far more competent wrecking corporation than any which tears down an old office building in a single week to make room for a parking place. On this twofold nature rests the whole valley strategy of the Department of Engineers. The river is their steam shovel, derrick, and hod carrier—a blind servant that works wonders if suggestions are discreetly conveyed to it; a sort of Caliban, if that be no libel. Its velocity, its burden of silt, and its broad valley dower it with a capacity to do things. Wherever the dikes parallel its shores, or cut across a chute, its slowed-down waters drop soil; the bank builds up, the chute dries up and then builds up, willows start, cottonwoods follow them, and in two or three years farmers are plowing in an old bed of the river. Wherever the dikes are thrust out from one shore toward the other, the latter backs off and the river comes in, and boats pass where a few years before red-winged blackbirds had been singing in the bushes.

There is more, of course. New banks, and old banks which are properly placed, are protected by stone revetments, often of hard red stone from South Dakota. Also a river bed is entitled to a mattress. These so-called mattresses further protect the banks, running out on the river bottom for half a hundred feet. There are thousands of them, woven from millions of the pliable young willow trees which spring up everywhere along the banks. I have seen great barges pass, piled high and four-square with willows, about as a hay wagon is piled with timothy when it starts down a rough lane for the farmer's barn. Weighted with stone, the mattresses quietly checkmate Caliban when, in tricky mood, he would undermine where he has builded.

Unlike the Ohio, the Missouri is not, nor ever can be in the section now being developed for navigation, a canalized river, with long pools between dams. Yet it has a number of canals. Pilot canals they are called, not because they guide pilots but because they guide the river. Upon decree that its bed should be changed, dredges cut a narrow channel through land on one side or the other. When the last "plug" of earth is removed from the head of the canal, the river sweeps in and begins to widen what man has started; its old bed shallows and then fills up, and on it in succession come the willows, cottonwoods, and farmers.

Fifteen minutes after one canal was opened, our pilot told me he had put his boat through; it went through in a hurry. There was drama in our own journey through the new channel, which was thirteen thousand feet long. The drama was enacted by a voice in the bow of the boat and reviewed by the rest of us up in the pilothouse. Soundings were incessant. They ranged from five feet, when there was but one foot of free water under us, to No Bottom, which was a plenty. The usual call that came up, however, was Mark Twain. I must have heard those words forty times. It occurred to me that Samuel L. Clemens was pretty smart in choosing a pen name for which a great American river provided incessant ballyhoo.

At the end of it all, the Missouri's canals will be un-recognized parts of its channel, its log picket fences will disappear under the silt, bushes and trees will cover them, and, in their ordered beauty, the river shores will be quite like those on the lower Ohio. That will be well, but it is not what the engineers are driving at. To some extent the old Missouri was—and to a less extent it is—not so much a river as just a route for water. The water flowed everywhere it pleased in a valley from two to seventeen miles wide. It followed secondary channels, it dissipated its volume in useless bayous, it flowed aimlessly through chutes behind sand bars. Every little while it played some scurvy trick, wiping out whole farms overnight or shifting them so that their title deeds are recorded in different counties, even in different states. For a minor illustra-tion, at De Witt Bend, sometimes called Box-Car Bend, I saw a string of old freight cars which a railroad had dumped into the water to protect its right of way against such a trespass.

Perhaps the river's meanest trick was to back away from
towns and leave them stranded miles inland. This it has
done fourteen times. In Glasgow where we spent a night
—we traveled only by day—I saw what it was about. It was
edging at various points into a neck of land, with the
purpose of cutting through, and leaving the town high
and dry, its railroad out of commission, and two great
river bridges spanning nothing but an ox-bow lake. The
engineers have forestalled that.

For such protective work the reason is obvious, but
why everything else that is being done? For answer, the
purpose is simply to turn a wide route for water into a
dependable river, keep it where it ought to be, and provide it with sufficient depths for navigation all the year
around, except in winter. At various times in its history
the Missouri has had its bed in every acre of land in a
valley that in places is seventeen miles wide. The plan is
to hold it between banks from seven hundred to eleven
hundred feet apart, letting it broaden out here and there,
particularly where tributaries come in. These tributaries,
however, must come in at an acute angle, and dikes have
been set up to see that they do; if they entered head foremost, the big river would slow them up and they would
drop their silt, forming bars. At the mouth of the Missouri the same thing is being contrived. Its channel has
been shifted downstream and contracted, so that the
mouth is little more than half as wide as older maps
show it.

The most interesting thing I learned on my voyage is
that water does not flow straight except through rocks,
and should not be asked to do so. As one of our party—
an unofficial member—put it, nature abhors a straight line.
It had always been my notion that the deepest part of a
river was the middle thereof, and that the bed was quite

like the tin gutter which runs along the eaves of a house. Not so, at least on the Missouri. The deepest water is found in the concave bends at either side. Was this caused perhaps by the rotation of the earth? My question brought out no answer more definite than "Oh, it's a way that water has."

Navigation on the Missouri is just a matter of following a concave bend until it begins to merge into a convex one and then moving over to the other shore and following a concave bend there until the same thing happens, when you return to the first side. The route you follow between the two concave bends is called a crossing. It is shallower there, but not so shallow as it is off the convex bends. If you followed a concave bend all the time, obviously you would travel in a circle and come back to where you started, and so would the river—which is not the way of rivers, though it is of lakes. Rivers have to go somewhere; lakes do not. Wherefore there must be convex bends, so that the river can get along. The pattern of concave-convex bends is that of the letter S.

A major object of Missouri River engineering is to see that proper concave bends are maintained and protected, are created where none exist, and corrected where too long or too short, or of irregular outline. There are also straightaways called reaches. It is not well that these should be very long. The longest, about seven miles and just above Pinckney Bend, is perhaps the most beautiful part of the river. Lofty bluffs clothed with hardwoods look down across the water from the left bank to a low-lying willow shore on the other side. The pilot said that in the fall these bluffs were something to see.

Where navigable water is provided on the Ohio by a series of dams with lock chambers for boats to pass, the same end is sought on the Missouri by collecting the flow in the bends of a narrowed channel. Because of its burden of silt, there may never be a dam upon it—save for the sections above those now being improved for navigation. If dams were set up in the navigable portions the river would drop its silt behind them, convert their pools into mere mudholes, and then flow over or around them. At Fort Peck, Montana, in the upper reaches of the river is a great new dam, the object of which is to store supplies for a reliable low-water flow down to the river's mouth. The lake which is collecting behind it will be two hundred feet deep at the dam-breast and will run back nearly two hundred miles. It should do a lot of good.

There are two other notable things about the Missouri. Where the Mississippi has hundreds of islands, its greatest western tributary has none, at least in the navigable section from Sioux City down. Formerly it had, and the names of some are on the maps. But they are all ex-islands except at high stages of the river. The chutes behind them were cut off because the main river had need of that water, and then the shore attached them to itself. The story of the Missouri is in its bends, the poetry is in their names. Here are some that attracted me: Dakota Bend, Winnebago, Black Bird, Little Sioux, Soldier, De Soto, Pigeon Creek, the Narrows, Council, St. Marys, Tobacco, Calumet, Nebraska, Otoe, Indian Cave, Arago, Rush Bottom, White Cloud, Squaw, Wolf Creek, Kickapoo, Bee Creek, Bean Lake, Contrary, Jackass, Sheep Nose, Fire Creek, Teteseau, Bon Homme, Slaughterhouse, Springhouse, Pelican, Plow Boy, Côte Sans Dessein Reach, South Point.

There is a separate story behind every one of these bends, but room here only for four. At South Point the Missouri reaches its farthest south. Because there were ladies aboard when a steamboat passed Jackass Bend, the

captain declared that it was Mule Bend. Somebody kept a
fine native wine in a springhouse overlooking Springhouse
Bend. Opposite another bend was a curious hill which
rose right out of the plain and was covered with trees and
grasses strange to the region. So the French called the hill
Côte Sans Dessein, which our pilot translated into "a Hill
without a Reason," ignoring my contention that it probably meant a shore without a pattern.

The other notable thing about the Missouri is that it
has two sets of levees, one of them home-made and seldom
in sight. I did not suspect its existence until the trip was
half over. When the farmers gained confidence in what
the government was doing, which was only two or three
years ago, and felt that the official banks would hold,
they began to raise earthworks of their own back in the
woods, to keep the flood water which got over the banks
from invading their fields. With one flood successfully
resisted, an earthwork would pay for itself. Some of the
earlier levees surrounded three sides of a farm. The later
plan was for neighbors to form levee districts and build
together. I was told that, except where there are bluffs,
these hidden enbankments follow both shores almost
down to the river's mouth.

Such was the present estate of the great stream I was
descending. Government had been working on it for
nearly a century, doing little beyond taking out snags
until the 1880's. Then the Missouri River Commission
was formed, made a study of channel regulation that has
been the guide for subsequent improvement, but never
received sufficient funds to do much. Its appropriations
had to be spent on revetments to protect valley property
rather than to improve navigation. In 1902 the Engineer
Department of the Army took over. In 1927 the project
assumed its present form, and adequate appropriations

accompanied it. About three years ago project plans were elaborated so as to pay closer attention to the creation of S-curves at the bends, to reduce the maintenance cost of dredging, to revet banks ahead of possible dangers, and to speed up the river's tasks of self-cleansing.

Perhaps the main change in objectives from the old days was in promoting navigation rather than in merely protecting shore property. The latter is still done where possible at waterworks intakes and bridges, even though this interferes with the best engineering practice. But the officers have no mandate to do anything except make the Missouri navigable. If one farmer finds himself possessed of a new meadow as a result of their moving the river away from his land and letting soil take the place of water, he is entitled to this accretion. If another farmer finds himself dispossessed of meadows because the river has been moved in on him, nothing can be done about it. Navigation is everything.

It has come into existence. Towboats and barges have been on the Missouri between Kansas City and its mouth since 1935. In 1938 more than half a million tons of commodities valued at over seventeen million dollars moved on this section of the river. In 1939 commercial navigation pushed upstream to Omaha, a large oil company making five trips thither from Kansas City, four of them being of four-barge tows, each with eight hundred thousand gallons of gasoline. Now there is some traffic as far up as Sioux City. This year's river tonnage is expected to double last year's. Commodities carried include vegetable products, chemicals, textiles, machinery, oil products, and vehicles shipped principally upstream, and grain and its products, feed, gasoline, clay, and steel-mill products shipped principally downstream.

I made a partial roundup of boats of all kinds upon the

river, most of which I saw. There are two Coast Guard cutters, the *Goldenrod* and the *Poplar;* two steamboats, the *Bixby* and *Suter;* the inspection boats, *Sergeant Pryor* and *Sergeant Floyd;* five great dredges; perhaps twenty gasoline launches of from one hundred to three hundred tons burden; twenty contractors' quarter boats; seven commercial towboats with their barge fleets, operated by the Inland Waterways Corporation, the Marquette Cement Company, and the Sioux City and New Orleans Barge Line; one showboat, the *Dixie Queen*. I made no count of various barges, some stacked with enough young willow trees to fill half a dozen haymows.

Through the years a lot of money has been expended in turning a wild river into a civilized waterway. When the task is complete the estimated cost will be $182,-000,000. Not counting navigation values, this outlay is practically halved by the indirect benefits to shore lands and other property. Nearly fifty million dollars has been added to the value of existing shore property by affording it security and protection from erosion. As an illustration, until two or three years ago, Omaha banks would not lend money on mortgage to a farmer whose land touched the river; they could not be sure that the farm would stay there, or even be anywhere. Now they lend. New and highly productive land has been reclaimed from the river bed. Its value is set at ten million dollars, a reasonable figure since the land amounts to perhaps a quarter-million acres. Furthermore, estimates show that maintenance expenditures formerly borne by the owners of waterworks, light plants, bridges, highways, railroads, and other public and private enterprises, in an effort to keep the river from moving in upon them, have been reduced by more than twenty-five million dollars. This makes a total of nearly eighty-six million dollars.

The other half of the nation's expenditure is repre-
sented by a river now restored to full commercial navigation as far up as Omaha, and approaching it as far up as
Sioux City. In a word, the six-foot channel which Congress decreed has actually come into being. That is not all.
In most cases the Missouri already has achieved more than
a six-foot channel, average depths being nearly double
that; and there is the great Fort Peck reservoir to draw
upon. For the expenditure of about six million dollars
more, in refinement work at the crossings, engineers say
that a nine-foot channel could be created, if Congress so
ordered. Then the Missouri's channel would have the
same minimum depth as the Ohio's and Mississippi's, and
boats of equal draft with theirs could ply upon it.

I have yet to speak of the army engineers in whose
charge is the Missouri and in whose company I made the
inspection trip from the head of navigation down to St.
Louis. Their chief is Colonel F. S. Besson, engineer for
the entire Missouri River Division, which has district
offices at Fort Peck, Omaha, and Kansas City; to his courtesy I am indebted for the fulfillment of a dream of long
standing. Two district engineers, Lieutenant Colonel Hel-
mar Swenholt of the Omaha office, and Major A. M.
Neilson of the Kansas City office, were also aboard. So
were Major John Arrowsmith, executive assistant to the
division engineer, and Major Francis H. Oxx, executive
assistant to the district engineer at Kansas City. We were
joined at different places, and upon another inspection
boat, by Captain Leland F. Wykert in command of the
Air Corps Detachment at Lincoln, Nebraska; Colonel
Jerome G. Pillow, army officer (retired) and Arkansas
planter; Arthur G. Everham, director of public works at
Kansas City; Willard J. Breidenthal, Kansas City banker,

and Guy E. Stanley, executive assistant of the Union Pacific Railroad.

The army engineers were a singularly interesting and of course a highly intelligent group. All had been places, serving their country in war and peace upon other waterways and in other lands: on the Ohio, on the Intra-Coastal Canal, in Cuba, in Japan, in the Philippines, and in the brief and nearly forgotten campaign against the Soviets in Arctic Russia. Their comradeship aboard was devoid of salutes and other ceremony, and at table I remarked a common fondness for such sincere American comestibles as corn pone, green onions, and the beverage known as milk.

After a while I became aware that some quality of drama invested this trip. A contact car accompanied us down the river, appearing at stated points to deliver or receive messages, to take off or put on officers, or just to disappear at a wave of dismissal from the pilothouse. This was routine and imperative on lonely river stretches, where the boat might break a shaft far from help or habitation. But the coming and going of the army engineers on our boat was not routine. None of them stayed long upon it. I went ashore with one to see what he was about—and fetched up at a huge, half-completed bomber plant at Fort Crook a few miles beyond Omaha. He was building it. It covers about fifteeen acres and will employ twenty-one thousand men, who will turn out Martin bombers. Other engineers of our group were building a bomber plant of about equal size at Kansas City, an airfield at Fort Riley, an airfield near Denver, an airport at Cheyenne, munition plants at various places.

Throughout state after state, in all the wide territory from which water flows toward the Missouri, these engineers are rearing defense works. At the same time they are watching the water, and with seeming ease carrying a double burden. At last I knew why the nation requires army engineers to do so much peacetime work on rivers— damming, dredging, revetting, straightening or twisting channels; commanding large work forces of their own, directing contractors with still larger forces under them. Thus are they schooled and disciplined for building munition factories, bridges, military roads, railroads, earthworks, and battle camps when war is on or near. Caliban, which is the Missouri, is a sort of college professor.

CHAPTER XXII

POPLAR SHORES

FOR the most part we moved through a world of willows and cottonwoods as we went down the Missouri. The willow is the most useful of all shore trees, springing up by the billions in chutes, in marshes, and in old beds of the river as soon as it goes elsewhere; making land also, and providing withes with which the unruly giant is bound down. The cottonwood or poplar, which is quite useless as lumber, is responsible for most of the snags in the channel; but it helps to make land, grows rapidly, and with its neighbors falls into stately processions along the river banks. It filled the air with its down as our boat went by, and I wondered why nobody had ever woven this into a fabric; it would make but a filmy garment, of course, yet perhaps all the better suited for models to wear at an Artists' Ball.

The characteristic fowl of the valley has the setting sun on its shoulders, the somber midnight as its tunic, and in its throat the wild sweetness of the first dawn song. This is the red-winged blackbird. Two other birds, however, are more numerous. One is the tern, flocks of which do their dipping food-dances over the water; it has no music save a thin cackle. I saw a white, beautiful, slant-rigged tern of a different species. The other bird which showed itself in numbers was the bank swallow, its twitter the mere ghost of a song. At one place were hundreds of nests in a cliff with the swallows hovering along its face or perched at the thresholds of their cave dwellings; Buffon would have called them troglodytes, which is no name for creatures so dainty. Out of every thicket where we stopped came the gay song of chewinks.

Among larger, cruder birds, I noted great blue herons patrolling the valley. Once at dawn I saw ten pelicans standing in conference in shallow water near the Nebraska shore. Later that morning a party of buzzards rose from some loathly but salutary banquet on a bayou's edge. Much of the time one of these large black birds was floating overhead. When a mudhen flew low across the water, information was volunteered that it was not bad eating if instead of plucking you skinned it, thereby divesting its carcass of an ancient and fish-like odor. Now and then a hawk dipped down into the bulrushes. Once a painted pheasant flew along a green alley of the wood. Crows were always alighting on the drift and seemed to prefer stumps; a good guess is that they were after grubs rather than a drink of Missouri River water, which, by the way, thick as it is, is quite potable. That is what—filtered of course— we drank on the boat.

The drift fascinated me. We overtook it at the mouth of the Platte, up which heavy rains had fallen. Daily we rode with it, got ahead of it, and then tied up for the night. In the morning it had overtaken us, and again for a while was our travel companion. It made the river look like a cornfield after husking time. The flotsam of other seasons, which floods had piled up on the log dikes, wrought outlandish effects. Sometimes it gave them the semblance of rude brush lodges thrown together by unskillful hunters. Stumps which were perched upon piles looked like giant bullfrogs. Trees wrapped themselves over the timbers like alligators climbing a fence. One trunk, couched along a dike, might have been a catamount about to spring. Colossal animals, saurians, extinct birds, the drift simulated them all. Its most striking piece of wooden sculpture was a blasted sycamore, too much like a skeleton lying on its back with sagging skull, sprawling limbs, and aimless fingers.

It was easy to fancy that on some night when there was no moon and few stars, but plenty of fox fire in the woods, these unhallowed forms might come to life and lead through the mists of the sleeping river a masquerade of days that were best forgotten.

These and kindred matters I pondered from the deck, where I spent all of my time except when in bed or at table or in the pilothouse. Missouri River winds are bluff but kind, and they and the warm sunshine did desirable things to me. One was to induce drowsiness between meals; but just when I nodded, in the middle of the forenoon or afternoon, along came the steward with a pot of coffee. Always I was conscious of an agreeable odor from the shore, where sweet clover grew wild. Sometimes there was mingled with this the scent of alfalfa hay curing in an upland field, of blooming catalpa trees down along the banks. The scene changed with every bend, little rivers entering, long sand bars appearing, jungles knotted together with wild grapevines coming and going, weedy bayous winding back to higher land, glimpses of russet wheat, yellow barley, gray-green rye, and pink plowed fields showing on distant farmsteads. Overhead white clouds formed and faded, only less substantial, I reflected, than shorelands which had been river bed before and would be such again.

Recognizing that I was a traveler and no student of navigation my shipmates volunteered items which they thought might entertain me. Did I know that you could train catfish? I did not. Yet the cooks on the quarter boats had done this thing. After meals they gathered up the scraps and banged on dishpans. Swarms of catfish as-

sembled for the feast. Another tale was so extraordinary
that I name the man who sponsored it, adding that I believed him. Major Arrowsmith told it, pinning it, I think,
on an uncle in Defiance County, Ohio. While this relative
was hunting with hounds, they treed some unusual crea-
ture, as their puzzled yelps proclaimed. Cautiously approaching a hollow sycamore, he peered into a hole and
found a large catfish in a pool of water, apparently thriving
on the grubs which infest such trees. High water had carried it inside and, receding, had imprisoned it.

There was also talk of beavers and wolves. I saw what
the former had been doing along the banks. In three or
four places they had cut down sizable trees, so as to feed
on the bark and tender shoots. One pilot reported that he
often saw a beaver perched on a dike gravely watching the
boat. An army engineer said that complaint had been
made to the Omaha office that these animals were cutting
down the finest shade trees at a summer camp, and what
was to be done about it? Nothing, for the law protects
them; and so in various sections they are returning to
their old haunts. The beaver created the fur trade, and
the fur trade opened up the continent. As much as the
buffalo, he is entitled to consideration.

One man said that on another trip he had seen a wolf
cross an open field and enter the woods. I was unaware
that there were wolves in Missouri, and suggested that
it might have been a coyote. But no, it was a timber wolf.
Farther downstream the wolf-legend took on the sub-
stance of reality. We passed the (ex) island of St. Aubert,
which is five miles long, a mile or so wide, and overrun
with rabbits. One of the crew, hunting with a friend, had
taken forty-eight in a single afternoon. Wolves favor rabbits and make forays upon the island from their dens in
the Ozark foothills which are just back of the river plain.

Nearly every farmer thereabout has a pack of wolf hounds. Hunts are organized, farmers riding to the known wolf crossings and waiting there for a shot. One old wolf has quite a reputation, at least among the hounds. When a pair of them get too far ahead of their fellows, he turns, disciplines them with claw and fang, and is off again. After that, they are still dogs but no longer hounds. Missouri pays bounties on wolf scalps.

Stopping at sunset instead of going on through the night was something new to me. Missouri River boats did that a hundred years ago, and people could get off and ramble around, if no Indian sign was noted. So I did. There are government lights from Omaha down for pilots to steer by, and commercial towboats travel at night; but as ours was an inspection trip that meant only daylight going. The first stop was at Omaha. I pass it up, because any city which has no better landing place for government officers— who are directing the expenditure of millions of dollars in that area—than a shabby, slippery ash heap, scarcely belongs in a travel narrative. I sprained a leg getting back to the boat.

Rulo was better. It may have four hundred inhabitants. I doubt if it is on any map. We stopped there in the late afternoon of the second day. Everybody got off and everybody else went away from there. I shifted to a companion boat, the *Sergeant Floyd*. Until nearly midnight I was its sole passenger. After Captain Henry Thomas, the master, had led me to my stateroom, and I had taken supper alone, I sat on the forward deck and watched the river rush by. It was going fast, perhaps six miles an hour, and had risen more than a foot since the previous evening. Word of my solitary estate may have reached the crew's quarters on the deck below. Anyway, the head of the boat's engineer— a veteran of the San Diego tuna fleet—showed above the

gangway. Would I like to see how the boys lived? On the
other boat I had merely surmised the existence of a crew.
This time I saw its members, sixteen strong, as well as
the glittering engine room beyond which were their quarters. They had shower baths and good bunks, and a large
messroom in which members were playing cards. A few
were taking showers, for something was doing ashore.

It seems that there is always something doing ashore
when a boat puts in at Rulo. When I went up the bank
and a hillside road to the hamlet to get sunburn ointment
and a few cards at the post office, I found out. There was
to be a dance that night in a new auditorium which was
also a gymnasium, admission twenty-five cents. I asked the
postmistress if it would be proper for a passing stranger
to attend and look on. She said it would.

As it was still daylight, I explored the village, first getting my bearings.

"Is this Iowa or Missouri?" I asked a native.

"Neither," he replied, "this is Nebraska."

I came across a bronze tablet set in a red sandstone
boulder which recited that Lewis and Clark had encamped
in 1804 at the foot of a cliff which could be seen from
there. After two days on the water familiar land things
seemed to have fresh appeal. Walking along I saw wayside
roses, iris, peonies, a potato patch in bloom. A column
of twittering swifts was pouring into a disused chimney,
wrens were bubbling, a dove mourning, a catbird spilling
snatches of remembered melodies in a twilight soliloquy.

In the dance hall on the hill, a young woman at the
door pinned on my coat a small square of orange paper,
perhaps a rain check. There was an orchestra of five pieces,
a crowd of fourscore persons of all ages. The postmistress
did not seem to remember my face, or she might have
been asked for a dance. I soon left, and hearing music on

the road back to the boat turned off and entered a tavern on the river bank. Dancing to a mechanical piano was going on in the barroom, and in the large dining room adjoining a party of men and women were eating fried chicken. Again I looked on. The tavern, I learned, had cottages to rent, was celebrated for its catfish dinners, and was—or planned to be—something of a resort. And that sums up all I heard about the little hamlet, except that there are a number of Indians in the country behind.

Returning to the vessel I put on a second pair of socks, for the night was chill, and sat up waiting for a group of men who were driving in from somewhere else. As its only visible occupant I felt that I should greet them, and I did. Pretty soon one of the officers said, "The boat is cold. We must have more heat." He went below. Then it dawned on me that I had welcomed him to his own boat.

At Kansas City, where we laid up for the third night, I was a casual spectator of a third dance, this one a sprightly sorority function with young girls in lovely long gowns and boys in white dress jackets. It was held on the roof of a clubhouse whence a citizen pointed out to me the course of the Kaw which comes in there, and which I wanted to see. In his car he took me through the old pioneer quarter to the noble and nobly placed World War memorial, and then out along the bluffs. The city has a very decent landing with a good flight of steps for government boats.

The Kaw was the second of two major tributaries of the Missouri, the mouths of which I had seen. At Plattsmouth, not far below Omaha, the Platte had come in, far narrower than I had expected and turbid from heavy storms. It is perhaps the best known of all unnavigable rivers; only Indians in bullboats drawing a few inches have ever made anything out of it. The main utilities of the Platte are for irrigation in the short grass country. Yet its mouth, as the

dividing line between the upper and lower Missouri, once
had a legendary repute, and passing it was celebrated by
Missouri River sailors as seamen still celebrate the crossing
of the Equator. Pawnees lived in its long valley, which
reached back through its two forks into the Rockies; great
herds of buffalo roamed there; the Forks of the Platte was
a geographical name of importance, and there were even
the Coasts of the Platte, which were low sand hills, far
from its mouth.

Because a great railroad runs up the valley, I have seen
something of the river. As I followed its course westward
through Nebraska, it was not always certain whether I
was looking at a river, a swamp populous with islands and
sand bars, or merely interlacing meadows on which a light
rain had fallen. However, I saw a large flock of wild geese
on one of the sand bars. The historical backgrounds are
as deep as the waters are shallow. Since the valley offers
an easy pathway to the foothills of the Rockies, early mov-
ers into the West preferred the route to any other. Over it
ran the Oregon Trail and its related pathways, the Mormon and the California Trails.

Although equally a broad and shallow waterway, the
Kaw, or Kansas, has a brief memory of steamboat navigation. This began propitiously with the trip of the *Excel* in
1854, bearing materials from Kansas City to build Fort
Riley, two hundred and forty miles upstream, or only
sixty miles below where the forks join to make the river.
Other low-water packets carried corn and passengers upon
it until the Civil War. Before the war closed, the Kansas
Legislature did what the railroads wanted it to do, declared the Kaw unnavigable, and authorized the building
of low-level bridges across it.

The Kansas-born Osage also has a memory of steamboats and in the Civil War of gunboats. After a meander-

ing journey of perhaps five hundred miles, it comes in at
Côte Sans Dessein some distance below Jefferson City,
the Missouri state capital. The river's other name is
Marais des Cygnes. Farther down we stopped at the mouth
of the Gasconade to get maps. Though its name carries
some echoes of boastful music, this is a well-behaved
waterway. It rises in the Missouri Ozarks and is three
hundred miles long; light-draught boats have ascended it
for a hundred. The mouth is used for a harbor and I saw
a great side-wheeler dredge lying in it. Here the Coast
Guard has a station, and the engineers a material yard and
a boat yard where major craft have been built. The black-
and-white buoys that mark one side of the Missouri's
channel are called Cans, and a glance tells you why. The
red-and-white buoys that mark the other side are called
Nuns, and I did not see why until I noticed a score of
them ranged beside a shed on the banks of the Gasconade.
They looked like a procession of nuns in red robes and
white-peaked caps pausing to say their devotions.

On the *Sergeant Floyd*, which was half again as large as
its sister boat and had the only texas I have ever seen
which passengers had not pre-empted, we went down
the river into a country where habitations were no longer
scarce. Mentally I dubbed the two commodious decks the
front porch and the back stoop. From them I saw historic
towns loom and fade—Independence, Leavenworth, Atchi-
son, St. Joseph—all jumping-off places for gold seekers and
settlers in another age. I scanned bluffs behind which were
reservations of those industrious farmers, the Omaha and
Winnebago Indians. In a dissolving panorama I saw the
valley world pass by—naked boys swimming in backwaters,
barefoot women waving from shanty boats, quarter boats
with the week's washing flying from their roofs, cattle
feeding in lush pasture fields, litters of small black pigs

with their dams perusing the flats, silver fireflies that were sunbeams dancing upon broken water. At half-hour intervals musical bells on the deck below proclaimed the time in sea-fashion; at four o'clock, eight, and twelve, eight bells sounded, and then the tale of the hours began again.

From time to time, shore or river matters, which may here be grouped, were made known to me. There is only one ferry on the Missouri from Sioux City down. Tabo, name of a former island, was once Terre Beau. On their westward exodus the Mormons crossed the Missouri a few miles above Omaha; a Mormon hill cemetery is on the Nebraska side. At Quindaro Landing fugitive slaves crossed into Free Kansas, biding for a space in a cave on the Kansas side. There has been recent rafting to a box factory in Mokane from timber lands fifty miles above. The Missouri town of Arrow Rock has a good Indian legend and a better steamboat hotel. Washington is the original home of commercial corncob pipes, known to the trade as Missouri meerschaums; special corn with thick cobs is grown thereabout and the cobs turned upon wooden lathes. The bluff towns—a good name—of Napoleon, Waterloo and Wellington almost adjoin each other.

Left to itself the Missouri, I was also told, will wash the sand out from under a boat stranded on a bar and set it free; to expedite their release, boats take spars along and practically walk out on stilts into deep water. In low water at the end of the navigation season, a snagboat goes up and down the river clearing out the logs. As the Missouri rises, crossings work downstream; they come up again when it drops. Two sets of mileage figures adjoining each other on the dikes and pilot lights give the distances from the mouth of the Missouri as of 1892 and 1930; sometimes they differ by as much as twenty miles—sign manual of a vagabond waterway.

On the last night we continued down the river until dusk, when we made fast to piles at the foot of a lonely bluff in a reach without a name. All I know is that it was fifty-one miles above Missouri's mouth. In the distance was the feeble flame of a lantern set out to guide passing boats. Stars came into the sky as darkness deepened, but to us there in the shadow of a steep and wooded shore they were of small avail. A wind sighed through the forest, crickets chirped, frogs put on their rhythmic hymn to night, or perhaps to love.

The four of us sat on the deck listening. Then a voice said, "I'm tired setting. Let's turn in." We did, and it was a little after eight o'clock on a night in May in the year nineteen hundred and forty-one.

Our vessel was under way before daybreak, as the river eased down into the lowland country, its long journey near an end. In the morning we passed a boathouse pavilion in a niche between white rocks. With its smokestacks and texas, almost it seemed to be a packet, and once it was. Part of it had come ashore to stay. When, an hour later, we entered the Father of Waters, a towboat with four barges crossed our course. It bore the only name possible for a boat to bear when the traveler comes out of the Missouri into the Mississippi and the boat is passing by. As the *Mark Twain* pushed on upstream its stern was a sheet of falling silver.

BIBLIOGRAPHICAL NOTES

Among the sources for background material as set forth below, the author makes special acknowledgment of the publications of the history departments of the State Universities of Iowa, Oklahoma, and Texas, and particularly of William J. Petersen's entertaining and authoritative account of steamboating on the Upper Mississippi, and the several volumes in which, with skill and scholarship, Grant Foreman has recalled to the country the dramatic but only dimly remembered land-and-water story of the American Southwest.

For the material availed of in bringing these chapters of river history up to the present and confirming and amplifying the author's personal observations, he acknowledges a major indebtedness to the annual reports of the Chief of Army Engineers and the several publications of the Corps of Army Engineers and its Ohio and Missouri River Divisions; to Documents of Congress, and to the publications of the United States Coast Guard, the Bureau of Fisheries, and the Bureau of Marine Navigation. The files of the *Waterways Journal* have again been of unique service.

ASBURY, HERBERT, *The French Quarter*.
AUGHINBAUGH, B. A., *Know Ohio*.

Baton Rouge Handbook.
BEADLE, JOHN H., *Western Wilds and the Men Who Redeem Them*.
BELTRAMI, GIACOMO CONSTANTINO, *A Pilgrimage in Europe and America*.

BRADBURY, JOHN, *Travels.*

BRITT, ALBERT, *Great Indian Chiefs.*

BULLETINS OF AMERICAN BUREAU OF SHIPPING, 1941.

BUREAU OF FISHERIES, Department of Commerce. Reports on mussel shells, pearls, meats, and buttons.

BUREAU OF MARINE NAVIGATION, *Pilot Rules for the Rivers Whose Waters Flow into the Gulf of Mexico.*

CABLE, GEORGE W., *The Grandissimes.*

CHAPPELL, PHIL E., *A History of the Missouri River.*

CHITTENDEN, HIRAM MARTIN, *History of Early Steamboat Navigation on the Mississippi.*

CINCINNATI *Times-Star,* Files.

CLEMENS, S. L., *Huckleberry Finn; Life on the Mississippi.*

COATES, ROBERT M., *The Outlaw Years.*

COOK, JIM (LANE) and T. M. PEARCE, *Lane of the Llano.*

CORPS OF ARMY ENGINEERS, *Improvement of the Missouri River.*

CRAMER, ZADOK, *The Navigator.*

CUMINGS, FORTESCUE, *Sketches of a Tour to the Western Country.*

CURTIS, GEORGE WILLIAM, *Orators and Addresses.*

DEATHERAGE, CHARLES P., *Steamboating on the Missouri River in the 'Sixties.*

DE BOW, J. D. B., "The Great Raft of the Red River and Its Removal," *De Bow's Commercial Review,* Vol. 19, 1855.

DE QUINCEY, THOMAS, *The English Mail Coach.*

DUNBAR, SEYMOUR, *A History of Travel in America.*

EGGLESTON, GEORGE CARY, *Recollections of a Varied Life.*

ESKEW, GARNETT LAIDLAW, *The Pageant of the Packets.*

FENNEMAN, NEVIN, *Physiography of the Eastern United States.*

FERBER, EDNA, *Show Boat.*

FISKE, JOHN, *The Mississippi Valley in the Civil War.*

FLINT, TIMOTHY, *Recollections of the Last Ten Years; Geography and History of the United States.*

FOREMAN, GRANT, *Adventure on Red River; Indian Removal; Marcy and the Gold Seekers;* "River Navigation in the Early Southwest," *Mississippi Valley Historical Review,* Vol. 15.

FREEMAN, LEWIS R., *Waterways of Westward Wandering.*

GARDINER, DOROTHY, *West of the River.*

GLAZIER, WILLARD, *Down the Great River.*

GOULD, E. W., *Fifty Years on the Mississippi.*

GRAYSON, FRANK Y., *Thrills of the Historic Ohio River.*

GREEN, ROBERT M., "The Conquest of the Llano Estacado," *Cincinnati Literary Club Papers.*

GREENBIE, MARJORIE BARSTOW, *American Saga.*

Greene Steamboat Newspaper, Vols. 1, 2, 3, 4.

GREGG, JOSIAH, *Commerce of the Prairies.*

GREVE, CHARLES THEODORE, *Centennial History of Cincinnati.*

HALL, JAMES, *Sketches of History, Life and Manners in the West.*

HANSON, JOSEPH MILLS, *The Conquest of the Missouri.*

HAY, JOHN, *Complete Poetical Works; Abraham Lincoln* in collaboration with John G. Nicolay.

HEARN, LAFCADIO, *Creole Sketches.*

HEMPSTEAD, FAY, *School History of Arkansas.*

HERBERT, VICTOR and HENRY BLOSSOM, *Mademoiselle Modiste.*

HERNDON, DALLAS T., *The Arkansas Handbook.*

HERODOTUS, *History.*

HOUSE DOCUMENTS, *Yazoo River, Miss. Document No. 198, 73d Congress, 2d Session; Red River, La., Ark., Okla. and Texas, Document No. 378, 74th Congress, 2d Session.*

ILLINOIS DEVELOPMENT COUNCIL, *Ten Tours in Illinois.*

IRELAN, JOHN ROBERT, *History of Zachary Taylor.*

JONES, ROBERT RALSTON, "The Ohio River," *United States Army Engineers Publication.*

KING, GRACE, *New Orleans, the Place and the People.*

LAUT, AGNES C., *The Blazed Trail of the Old Frontier.*

LIGHTY, KENT and MARGARET, *Shanty-Boat.*

LONG, STEPHEN H., "Expedition to the Rocky Mountains," *Early Western Travels.*

LONGFELLOW, HENRY WADSWORTH, *Evangeline.*

LOUISIANA TOURIST BULLETIN, Vol. 3, No. 8 (8).

LOUISIANA TOURIST BUREAU, *This is Louisiana.*

LUDWIG, EMIL, *The Nile: the Life Story of a River.*

New Orleans City Guide, WPA Federal Writers Project.
NEWELL, GEORGIE WILLSON and CHARLES CROMARTIE COMPTON, *Natchez and the Pilgrimage.*
NUTTALL, THOMAS, *A Journal of Travels Into the Arkansas Territory.*

OHIO RIVER DIVISION, CORPS OF ARMY ENGINEERS, *Dredging Technique; Navigation on the Ohio River.*

PARKMAN, FRANCIS, *The Oregon Trail.*
PETERSEN, WILLIAM J., *Steamboating on the Upper Mississippi.*
PLUTARCH, *Lives.*

ROOSEVELT, THEODORE, *The Winning of the West.*
RUSSELL, CHARLES EDWARD, *A-Rafting on the Mississip.*

SAXON, LYLE, *Father Mississippi.*
SCHIERLOH, SAMUEL, *Grains That the Huskers Lost.*
SEITZ, DON C., *Uncommon Americans.*
SELLARDS, E. H., B. C. THORP and R. T. HILL, "Investigation on the Red River, Made in Connection with the Oklahoma-Texas Boundary Suit," *University of Texas Bulletin,* July, 1923.
SEMPLE, ELLEN CHURCHILL, *Influences of Geographic Environment.*
SHAKESPEARE, WILLIAM, *Antony and Cleopatra.*

TOUSLEY, ALBERT S., *Where Goes the River.*

UNITED STATES ARMY ENGINEERS, *The Middle and Upper Mississippi River; Report upon the Improvement of Rivers and Harbors in the Vicksburg, Miss., District; Report on the Yazoo River; Nov. 1933; Annual Reports.*
UNITED STATES COAST GUARD, *Light List on Ohio and Mississippi Rivers.*

Waterways Journal, Files.
WILSON, CHARLES E., *History of Coles County.*
WRIGHT, DONALD T., *Diary of a Steamboat Trip up the Arkansas.*

INDEX

J

Jackson, Andrew, 65, 94
John Ordway, 221-224

K

Kanawha River, 121
Kansas City, 248
Kansas River, 249
Kaskaskia, 111, 146, 148, 150-151
Kaskaskia River, 148-149
Kaw River, 248
Kentucky meals, 138
Kentucky River, 22, 121

L

Lafayette, Marquis de, 17
Lafitte, Jean, 65
Law, John, 89
Lead mining, 201-202
Lee, Robert E., 133-134
Leech River, 143
Levees, 236
Lewis and Clarke Expedition, 224, 247
Leyhe, Captain W. H. "Buck," 158, 161
Licking River, 22
Life on the Mississippi, 173
Little Hocking River, 140
Little Kanawha River, 121, 140
Little Miami River, 22
Little Muskingum River, 140
Llano Estacado, 79-81

Loggy Bayou, 77
Longfellow, Henry Wadsworth, 46
Louisiana Purchase, 85, 224
Louisiana, slave code of, 66
Louisville, 17
Lumber camps, 207
Lumbering, 206-209

M

Mackenzie, General, 80
Mademoiselle Modiste, 172
Marais des Cygnes River, 250
Marcy, Captain Randolph B., 78, 85
Mardi Gras, 73-74
Marine Insurance, 122-124
Martin's Ferry, 141
McKenzie, Kenneth, 225
Memphis, 33
Migration of Five Civilized Tribes, 92-98
Minnesota River, 203, 216
Mississippi Bubble, 31
Mississippi River, 28-35, 111
Mississippi River locks, 166, 183-184, 186-187, 194-195
Mississippi River, Lower, 107, 143
Mississippi River, Middle, 15, 143
Mississippi River, Upper, 15, 143, 178-184, 187
Missouri River, 15, 143, 171, 219-220, 221, 228-241

37
4/72

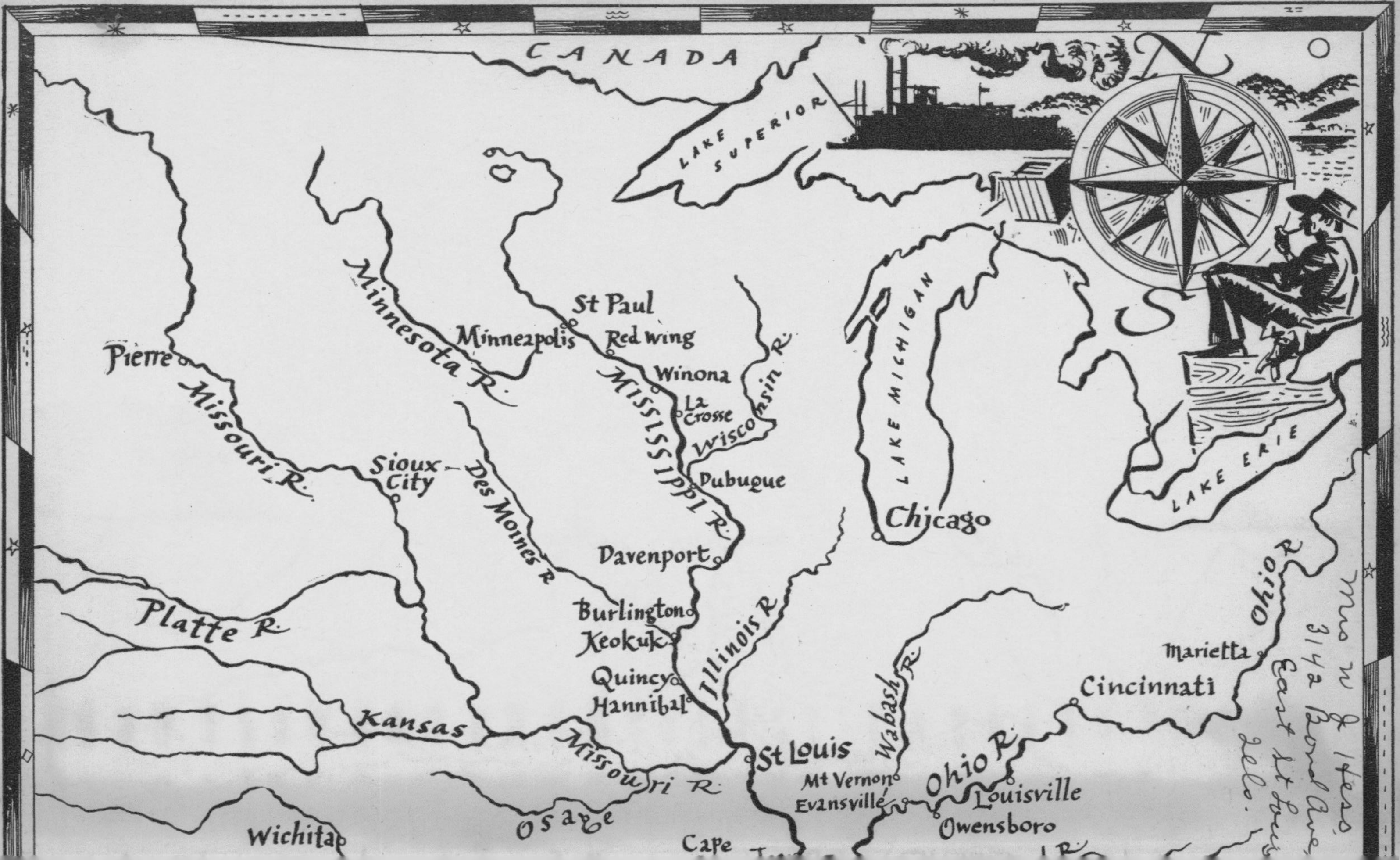
CANADA
LAKE SUPERIOR
N
S
LAKE MICHIGAN
LAKE ERIE
St Paul
Minneapolis
Red wing
Winona
La Crosse
Wisconsin R.
Dubuque
MISSISSIPPI R.
Minnesota R.
Pierre
Missouri R.
Sioux City
Des Moines R
Davenport
Burlington
Keokuk
Quincy
Hannibal
Illinois R.
Chicago
Platte R.
Kansas
Missouri R.
Osage
Wichita
Cape
St Louis
Wabash R.
Mt Vernon
Evansville
Ohio R.
Louisville
Owensboro
Cincinnati
Marietta
Ohio R.
Mrs W J Hess
3142 Bond Ave,
East St Louis
Ills.